Eat and Relax

The Only Way to Permanent Normal Weight and Good Health

By Kelly Jones

This book is dedicated to everyone that I have known and loved, who like me, have struggled with eating disorders, weight and health.

Table of Contents

REFERENCES

Introduction

This is a personal story. Nothing here should be misconstrued as medical advice. I believe, however, that there are some universal truths in it. Some things that seem to be universally true are: Everyone wants to be in good health. Everyone believes that there is a body weight that equates to good health. Everyone wants to have the energy to do the things that they want to do. Everyone wants to be considered attractive to others. Everyone thinks that if they could achieve a desirable weight, they would be, not only attractive to others but energetic and happy, as well. Almost no one knows how to achieve and keep an optimal weight and also have good health.

Where weight is concerned, there are certain things that the vast majority of people in the world believe. Some of these beliefs are:
1. If a person eats "too much" they will get fat.
2. If a person wants to lower their weight they must lower their caloric intake and exercise more.

3. It is the excess weight that a person carries that "causes" negative health conditions, like diabetes, heart problems, cancer and stress on the joints.

4. If a person is at the weight that a Body Mass Index {BMI) chart deems to be in the normal range, regardless of what they are doing to be at that weight, that person will be healthier than those in the overweight or obese ranges.

5. The problem of obesity in the populace can be laid at the door of too much "highly palatable", refined food availability.

I used to believe those things too. I have proved to myself that they are not true. In talking about weight, I am going to describe what is desirable for each individual as "normal weight". No number can be put to what is normal that would be true for everyone. No percentage of body fat can be used. Normal is different for each individual. The word "normal" stands in for the particular weight span at which a given individual will be the healthiest. It is true that not everyone thinks of the same thing when they are picturing someone they would consider to be at a "normal" weight. Some people picture anything but a normal weight when it comes to what they want for themselves, often picturing themselves at a weight that would be significantly under their normal weight. I will use the word "normal" for the ideal weight that each individual can achieve. I will use no external metrics, such as BMI charts, to idealize the weight that is desirable for anyone, for reasons I will later explain. I will use the word "obesity" only in the context of public health concerns. I will use the expression "excess fat" to describe a biological reality with no moral judgment attached to the term.

Reasonably, people want a normal weight, but it seems to be increasingly difficult to achieve. I have observed, in my lifetime, the growing struggle to maintain an optimal weight among the American populace and the export around the world of this problem. Animals that are in charge of their own food intake, always have the normal fat deposition for their species, provided that there is no famine, varying with the time of year. Why have humans entered an unprecedented time of difficulty maintaining the various normal body shapes that are natural to us? I am sure you think you know the answers to this question. You have been listening to the ideas posited from media sources and in your doctor's office or gym, which I listed above. Everyone has been hearing the same message over and over, but what has that information achieved except a worsening problem? It is being called a catastrophe of epic proportions. Obesity is being spoken of as a major contributor to negative outcomes during the SARS-CoV-2 pandemic. Pundits, concerned with the connection between negative outcomes from Sars-CoV-2 infections and obesity, blithely state that people need to lose weight. They complain, rationally, about the injunctions against going outside and getting some exercise during the pandemic, as counterproductive to good health. They ignore the fact that none of the measures recommended by the mass of advisors has ever worked to keep excess fat off of our bodies. Everyone is concerned, but the concern has not been able to come up with one sure-fire way to permanently beat excess fat, and at the same time bring about vibrant health, which must include immune systems that work as they should.

I've been concerned about myself, my family and everyone else. That concern has led me on a thirty-nine year search for answers. For all of those years, I have been very interested in health issues and how to achieve better health through nutrition. I have gone deeper and deeper into the research of nutrition, health and weight and the place where these concepts meet. When I was raising my kids, I decided I wanted to take some distance courses from the Natural Healing Institute of Naturopathy in Encinitas, California. Through that school, I qualified as a Certified Clinical Nutritionist. My self-propelled education has continued since that time, because by no means, had I gotten to the bottom of the troubles that continued to afflict my own health and that of others at the end of my course. My continued search has paid off. I have been able to achieve a normal weight and a reversal of all of the negative health conditions that had accumulated, but only in the last five years. Even though I was qualified, for many years in a technical sense, to teach others about how nutrition impacts health, I never felt that I really had found the answers I was looking for, though I was trying many things and talking about them while I was learning. My own health had been worsening during that time and I did not know, in spite of all of my studies, how to achieve stable weight. In time, that changed, as a result of continued research. I am grateful to have found the answer, with the help of many other researchers who "were onto something". In piecing all of these various scientific findings together, I found something that I was convinced would work and that I was willing to try on myself. I am glad that I did. I am going to share my experience here.

Here is a list of ways, often recommended, that are supposed to help a person shed pounds. You have been hearing about and trying these things. I have tried all but four of them and they did not bring about a permanent state of normal weight or good health for me. In no particular order they are:

1. Cutting calories

2. Avoiding carbohydrates

3. Exercising more

4. Eating "carnivore"

5. Eating paleo

6. Raw meat diet (version of "carnivore")

7. Low-fat diet

8. Intermittent fasting

9. Skipping meals

10. Portion control

11. Food combining principles

12. Gluten-free diet

13. Any variety of fasting

14. Eliminating any particular food from the diet

15. Including some particular food in the diet, except for a broad category like carbohydrate

16. Chewing thirty times

17. Eating nothing after 7 p.m., or any other time of night

18. Avoiding sugar

19. Vegan diet

20. Avoiding any "white" food

21. Putting our fork down between bites

22. Serving our meal on a smaller plate

23. Drinking water only

24. Avoiding snacking

25. Attending any kind of weight-loss program, whether in person or online

26. Being a contestant on any television show for weight-loss purposes

27. Any kind of surgery, like gastric-bypass

28. Eating "clean"

29. Eating "all natural"

30. Eating raw

31. Purging

32. Giving ourselves twenty minutes to digest before taking a second helping

33. Ketogenic diet

34. Chorionic Gonadotropin Diet

35. The "French woman's" diet

This book will explain why I say, categorically, that none of these things will bring about permanent normal weight or good health. Please note, the operative word is "permanent". In the first chapter, I will explain what I mean by permanent weight loss and good health.

Chapter 1

If I Can Gain Weight I Am Doing It Wrong

A permanent state of normal weight, along with good health, is possible. Extreme old age will come but, in between now and then, there are many variables. We have choices to make which will impact the ability of the living organism, which is our body, to maintain good health. Excess fat on a body is a symptom, often but not always, seen with other symptoms of a struggling organism. It is a symptom of adjustments the body is having to make to cope with what is being done to it. Along with this symptom, of a body that is coping with the environment it is in, are other symptoms that have become prevalent. Auto-immune disorders, osteoporosis, arthritis, eye issues, cardiac issues. vascular troubles, Parkinson's disease, cancer, metabolic issues and so forth, have become common where I live, in the United States. We are not to blame for these things affecting our health, because information about how to maintain normal weight and good health has been heavily obscured by misguided ideas and a system of scientific research which keeps scientists, from different disciplines, from effectively coalescing their findings. The information is all there, but how to plow through the thousands of research papers and studies? For the year 2020, the number of new citations added to PubMed is listed as 362,528. That is a lot of material to research. To add to the difficulty, when I read some studies, it is clear from the Summary section, that the researchers are trying to make the data gathered fit a pre-existing notion. Of course, we all have confirmation bias, but I have realized that I cannot confine myself to reading just the conclusion of an article. No one should feel badly about not figuring out how to really help themselves stabilize their weight and enjoy good health when it is so difficult. Doctors want stable weight and good health, too, but they are just very busy people who only know what they know. Their job is to help us and they want to, but nutrition is rarely taught in medical schools. If it is taught at all, it is only a few hours of instruction in a body of research that is as complicated as the proverbial "rocket science". They are no more likely to give good advice on this subject than anyone else who has read Men's Health magazine. Of course, we consult our doctors when we have an issue, and we receive palliatives to help us cope with what is bothering us. However, where achieving normal weight forever is concerned, nothing has helped. Also, let's face it, there are interests in this world not served by solving the obesity problem. Keeping us in a state of anxiety about our weight and fueling an interest in spending money fruitlessly on the problem serves such interests much better.

I am going to make a bold statement, which I know to be true. This is the main tenet of this book. It is the goal, concerning weight, that I have reached since implementing what I now understand about human biology. Along with reaching this weight goal, I have also seen every health problem I had previously been experiencing reversed. The statement is, the only way to really know that I am doing the right thing where my dietary intake is concerned is to have reached the point where I do not gain weight, no matter how much I eat.

That is right. How do I know that is right? Because after thoroughly researching the subject for more than thirty-five years, I finally saw what the science was saying and I tried the method that emerged from that research. After decades of constant and frustrating fluctuation of my weight and the accumulation of symptoms of ill-health, I am now in the place I hoped to be. I do not gain weight, no matter how much I eat, period. This has been the case for over four years. I know it is right because I practice my research findings every day. I know it is right because, even during the current pandemic, when I observe that so many have experienced it as a time of weight gain, I have not gained weight. It is very freeing to be in this state, because I can simply enjoy my food and not worry about my body, at all. I think it would be a great thing if everyone could be in that place. I also feel that it would be wonderful if everyone could experience the reversal of health conditions that I see they are suffering from, just as I was, but no longer experience. Good health is the body being able to repair the things that become damaged, in the course of normal life. It is a body that is able to perform all normal functions. It is a body with an immune system that functions properly. That does not mean that a person does not get a virus. It means that the immune system handles the virus properly.

After I began to implement my findings, I searched to see if anyone else was doing the things I was doing. I found some. From that I learned that I was not just an "N=1 experiment". That is also how I know that the above statement about weight gain is right. I wonder who else is absolutely confident that they can eat any amount of food that they feel like eating, without putting on any weight. Probably those who are just doing that every day without thinking about it much. We all know them. They just eat and they are healthier and thinner than anyone else we know. I found out that eating as much as I want, at any time, of anything that I feel like eating, is how I am getting everything that my body needs to maintain good health. It often strikes me that zebras, on the Serengeti plain, eat everything they want every day without putting on excess fat, but humans cannot manage it. We cannot do the most basic thing, feed ourselves, without getting ourselves into trouble. It is our tendency to intellectualize everything that is the problem. Zebras do not do that. Nor do any others who share this planet with us do that. Some of the people we know are like that, too. A few others have found the research that I found and have had the same results as I have had,, a return to normal weight and a reversal of negative health issues. "Normal weight" is what animals can achieve, but too few humans know how.

There are processes that happen in our bodies every day that we do not have to think about. They happen automatically. However, we want to learn about what is going on with our bodies, because we are curious and we want to understand. That is natural. The problem is, we are arrogant. We think we know enough at any given time, to start using our intellects to manipulate things in our bodies. Processes that have been going on for as long as there have been human bodies, without manipulations, can now be measured, judged and "improved" upon, so we think. We survived and even thrived, in various places on earth, for millennia, without intervention, eating the various foods available in the particular locale. However, now that we know about calories and nutrients and hormones and how to measure bodily processes, we think we know enough to start tinkering. It has been to our detriment. I, certainly, was not benefited physically by the knowledge that I had garnered from many years of study, until, finally, I was. It is not the search for knowledge that is the problem. It is the assumption that at any given moment we know enough to start doing some extreme things to our bodies. What I am talking about is the opposite of manipulating and forcing our bodies. I will explain in what ways we have been mistaken and have been treating our bodies badly, with the realization that the fullest explanation would require many books.

Chapter 2

Tried At My Own Risk

I will group some of the items, from the list in the introduction, that I said would not lead to permanent weight loss and good health and explain why I say that. I will begin with:

-Chorionic Gonadotropin Diet

-"French Women's Diet"

-Cutting calories

-Portion control

-Low-fat diet

-Skipping meals

-Any variety of fasting

-Eating nothing after 7 p.m., or any other time of night

-Putting our fork down between bites

-Serving the meal on a smaller plate

-Drinking water only

-Not snacking

-Attending any kind of weight loss program whether in person or online

-Any kind of surgery, like gastric-bypass

-Purging

-Giving ourselves twenty minutes to digest, before taking a second helping

The basic principle upon which all of these diets or practices supposedly works is the idea that weight gain is a matter of the consumption of too many calories. Consume fewer calories, the reasoning goes, and voila, the body must use its own fat for energy and a person will lose weight. Everyone talks about this like it is obvious. Most think of any calories that we do not immediately "burn off" by exercising as energy that will be stored as fat. It seems very logical to just cut calories. "The fewer, the better" seems to be everyone's view. All of the above practices are recommended by someone, because they will force or trick a person into consuming fewer calories.

Most weight loss programs are designed to apply a metric to the consumption of food, so that we can more easily avoid calories. In spite of the fact that advertisements say that HCG[1] (Human Chorionic Gonadotropin hormone) will "attack fat" and "eliminate cravings", it is the very low calorie diet of 500 calories per day that causes the rapid weight loss. The lack of hunger that those who have been on the diet say they experience is caused by the body entering ketosis and using its own tissue for energy, both fat and muscle. Gastric-bypass surgeries force a minute intake of food by creating a small pouch at the top of the stomach that can only hold one ounce of food. This pouch is then attached to the middle of the small intestine which means that fewer calories are absorbed. Most bariatric surgeries also divide the vagus nerve, which regulates the digestive

---

[1] Rabe T, Richter S, Kiesel L, Runnebaum B; Risk-Benefit Analysis of a hCG-500kcal Reducing Diet (cura romana) in Females; 1987 May; "Four out of 10 studies with negative results were controlled studies (hCG vs. control without hCG), whereas 6 were double-blind studies. These studies showed a significant weight reduction during dieting, but no differences between treatment groups in respect of body weight, body proportions and feeling of hunger. One of them is the only German study conducted by Rabe et al. in 1981 in which 82 randomized premenopausal volunteers had been dieting either with hCG or without hCG injections. In recent publications describing mostly well-documented double-blind studies authors largely reject hCG administration in dieting. Supporters of the hCG diet must prove the efficacy of this method in controlled studies according to the German Drug Law. Until then the opinion of the German steroid toxicology panel is still valid, that hCG is ineffective in dieting and should not be used."

system's response to carbohydrate. Vomiting (purging) food allows no time for normal utilization of calories to occur. The usual explanations given about how French women remain very slim center around portion control with occasional fat avoidance. Snacking is also discouraged in French culture. It all adds up to limiting calories. French women who do these things are not fat proof. If they give up calorie limiting practices, they will gain weight. Can anyone lose weight doing any of these things? Yes. It is true that, if anyone suddenly reduces caloric intake, their body, accustomed as it is to a certain metabolic rate based on the amount of calories they have been eating, will be forced to use some of its own tissue to make up for the shortfall. The metabolic rate will soon be lowered, however, by stopping or slowing down processes and curtailing repairs, so that the body does not quickly use itself up[2]. Can anyone keep excess weight off permanently doing any of these things? No, and especially not if they want to be well. I will explain, in the next chapter, why these manipulations cannot ever lead to permanent weight loss along with good health.

---

[2] Mole PA; Impact of Energy Intake and Exercise on Resting Metabolic Rate; Sports Med, 1990 August 10; "Resting metabolic rate is measured by the amount of calories consumed in the diet relative to energy expenditure. Excessive consumption of energy appears to increase resting metabolic rate while fasting and very low calorie dieting causes resting metabolic rate to decrease. Since the metabolic rate at rest is the primary component of daily energy expenditure, its reduction with caloric restriction makes it difficult for obese individuals to lose weight and to maintain weight that is lost."

For now, I will group a couple of other items from our list:

-Exercising more

-Being a contestant on any television show for weight-loss purposes

Exercise is presented as the most bog-standard addition to calorie reduction for weight-loss purposes. It is, supposedly, the least extreme thing presented as the solution to all of our weight problems. The idea of "eat less and exercise more" is ubiquitous in the media offering advice to the populace concerning their expanding waistlines. Also to be considered is that exercise increases our metabolic rate temporarily, therefore leading to weight loss, so we are told. So, the message that is being delivered as to why we are gaining so much fat is that we are too lazy and gluttonous. In so far as a television reality show is based on the idea of cutting calories and increasing exercise for the purpose of bringing about weight loss, it belongs in this grouping. Can anyone lose weight by beginning a program of increased exercise? Yes. Will the weight loss be permanent? No. Exercise is another way of cutting calories. The fuel that someone takes into their body that must be used to energize a workout is fuel not available for body processes and repairs. There are health benefits to getting out in the fresh air and sunshine and to moving our bodies, but any weight loss effects that occur from suddenly increasing the time spent exercising or the intensity of our exercise, will be temporary[3]. I will speak more about exercise in chapter 7.

Another grouping from our list is:

-Avoiding carbohydrates

-Eating Paleo

-Eating "carnivore"

-Avoiding sugar

-Avoiding any "white" food

-Ketogenic diet

One of the ideas behind these modifications is the avoidance of carbohydrates, or certain carbohydrates in the diet. Carbohydrate is one of the three macronutrients in our food. Along with carbohydrates, are protein and fat. Stating the obvious, they are all three nutrients and therefore nutritious for us to consume. Every one of these macronutrients are vilified by some practitioners of some of the items in the master list, in the introduction. Recently, carbohydrates have been the target for control by many of these diets. The "avoid 'white' food" idea is about refined

---

[3] Westerterp Klaas, Exercise, Energy Balance, and Body Composition; European Journal of Clinical Nutrition 2018 September 5; "Fat loss over 10 months was not much larger than fat loss over the similar 3-month intervention of the earlier study described above. Thus, individual responses of exercise training on energy balance and body composition in overweight and obese subjects are highly variable and reach a plateau in time."

carbohydrate, yes, but also about avoiding potatoes along with white rice, sugar and refined flour. The proponents of Paleo diets end up avoiding many carbohydrate sources since they practice avoiding any of the foods from agriculture, like grains and sugar. The idea behind all of these diets is that carbohydrate is somehow an especially bad food for humans. Avoiding it will allow bodies to work properly, the theory goes, and it is the idea, to a large extent, behind the glycemic index. The effect of some carbohydrates to raise the blood sugar level more quickly is what is being measured to form the index, and the faster a food raises blood glucose, the more damaging it is supposed to be. It is sometimes this idea that carbohydrates cause diabetes that contributes to their status as something to avoid, in the eyes of many. It has been my observation, however, that what happens to the promoters of low carbohydrate diets of many varieties is that, over time, they develop diabetes. This needs to be examined and the mechanism understood. Can a person lose weight by changing their current diet to any of these diets? Yes. Will it lead to permanent weight loss and good health? No.

We will move on to other macronutrient-avoidant diets like:
-Vegan
-Raw vegan

Eating raw is usually a more extreme version of being vegan, though some follow a raw meat diet. All food would be uncooked in this variation of veganism. Vegans avoid all food sources from something "with a face", as I have often heard it explained. Honey, coming from bees, qualifies as a food they avoid. Maple syrup coming, as it does, from trees, which have no face, is a food that would not be avoided by a vegan. Vegans avoid animal protein, but derive protein from plant foods. Weight loss is not, usually, the primary reason anyone takes up a vegan diet, but it is often touted as a benefit. Some thought has to be given to complete proteins in the diet as, along with the meat of an animal, dairy and eggs are avoided. These foods contain complete proteins, which beans, a vegetable protein source, for example, do not. It is a lot easier to fall into a below par protein state in the body for a vegan, than it is for someone who eats meat, or who is an ovo-lacto vegetarian (someone who eats eggs and dairy products, as well as plant sources of food[4]). If someone adopts any version of veganism, can they lose weight? Yes. Can they maintain any weight loss and enjoy long

[4] Marzola, Nasser, Hashim, et al; Nutritional Rehabilitation in Anorexia Nervosa: Review of the Literature and Implications for Treatment; BMC Psychiatry 2013, November 7; "Patients with AN tend to consume vegetarian diets more often than the general population.....their diet results in low calorie and low fat meals, insufficient for daily calorie, essential fatty acid, and amino acid requirements."

term good health, too? Not if avoiding food from "anything with a face" is their only concern.

Another classic avoidant diet is:

-Low-fat diet

I included this in the calorie-avoidant group, as well, because it is usually the main macronutrient limited in those kinds of diets where caloric intake is viewed as the essential problem to be solved. Both carbohydrates and proteins contain 4 calories per gram, whereas fat contains 9 calories per gram. So, to limit fat in the diet is a logical strategy to limit calories. In the public mind, however, there is also a notion that the fat we consume goes most directly to fat storage in the body. The biology of what happens to food, once it is consumed, is not as simple as that, however. More recently, paleo and ketogenic diets promote fat as healthful for the body. The ability to enter into ketosis relies on limiting carbohydrate and to a lesser extent protein, so fat is emphasized in diets like Atkins, Carbohydrate Addicts and what is simply called "keto". It is in diets like Pritikin and Ornish, named after their creators, that low-fat eating is glorified. Can anyone lose weight if they begin a low-fat diet? Yes. Can the weight-loss be maintained along with good health? Not if keeping fat low in the diet is the only concern[5].

---

[5] Lichtenstein Alice, Van Horn Linda; Very Low Fat Diets AHA Journals 1 September 1998 "Investigators warn that subjects frequently adjust to the

How about practices advocated by some magazines and in online commercials like:

-Eating "clean"

-Eating "all natural"

-Eliminating any particular food from the diet

-Including some particular food in the diet, (with the exception of a broad category, like carbohydrate)

All of these ideas have the belief, at bottom, that there is something in a particular food that can sabotage weight loss efforts or enhance weight loss. The premise behind "clean" eating is that food should be as close to nature as possible. Minimally processed is what someone is looking for here. And "all natural" is really the same. There is no end of particular foods, suggested by someone or other, to either include or eliminate from the diet, in order to create conditions favoring weight loss. Everything from certain fruits, vegetables, meats, seafood, fats and broader categories which I have discussed already are recommended by someone for inclusion or exclusion. The recommendations center on some constituents of these foods which are deemed to either positively or negatively impact individual

---

low-fat regimen over longer periods of time and increase energy intake, sometimes to prestudy levels. Under less restrained conditions, individuals compensate for alterations in the macronutrient content of the diet."

health and weight. Diets such as those based on the ancient medical practice of Ayurveda and The Blood Type Diet heavily use this idea, based on factors of individual uniqueness.

Can a person lose weight by eliminating or including some particular food in the diet (except in the instance of including back in a broad category, such as carbohydrate)? Yes. Will this be permanent? No. Not if that is all that person is doing. Most people who see weight loss from doing something along these lines, are combining the elimination or inclusion with some kind of calorie avoidance, either deliberately or accidentally.

A special category of food avoidance we must include with the elimination category is:

-Avoiding gluten

This measure is palliative for many people (palliative, too, can be the elimination of some other foods, but not curative). Avoiding gluten is life-saving for those who have an autoimmune response to gluten. Those with celiac disease must avoid gluten. It has become common for those without celiac disease to avoid gluten when they experience gastrointestinal symptoms or a wide variety of other symptoms which are blamed on gluten, which is a protein that some grains contain. Can an individual lose weight by eating only foods that are gluten-free? Yes. Will that change achieve relief from the symptoms being experienced?

Sometimes. Will any weight loss from making such a change be permanent? No. Will the problem causing the symptoms be cured? The actual cause of the problem has not been addressed, so no. Can anyone stave off health problems from ever occurring by the preemptive avoidance of gluten-containing foods? No[6].

Some other practices are:

-Food-combining principles

-Eating raw[7]

---

[6] Biesiekierski J, Peters S, Newnham E, Rosella Q, Muir J, Gibson P; No Effects of Gluten with Self-Reported Non-Celiac Gluten Sensitivity After Reduction of Fermentable, Poorly Absorbed Short-Chain Carbohydrates; Gastroenterology May 6, 2013 "Generally NCGS is viewed as a defined illness, much like celiac disease, where gluten is the cause and trigger for symptoms. In such a case, it would be anticipated that removal of gluten from the diet would lead to minimal symptoms and subsequent exposure to gluten would lead to specific triggering of symptoms. The results of the current study have not supported this concept....in 2 randomized, double-blind, placebo-controlled, cross-over trials specific and reproducible induction of symptoms with gluten could not be demonstrated."

[7] Cottier, Cody; Cooked Veggies Are Often More Nutritious Than Raw. Here's Why; Discover December 11, 2020 "experts say that more often than not, the opposite is true: Cooking unlocks the health benefits of many plants.....the British Dietetic Association named the raw vegan diet one of the five "celebrity diets to avoid" in 2018, noting that many foods are more nutritious after cooking. 'The human body can digest and be nourished by both raw and cooked foods,' the association wrote, so there's no reason to believe raw is inherently better"

-Raw carnivore[8]

-Chewing thirty times

These belong with the previous, in a way. The thing that you would be adding into the diet are more nutrients, the theory goes. Food combining principles and chewing thirty times supposedly aid the most complete digestion and nutrient utilization of all of our meals. Eating raw food supposedly helps, by not cooking out the nutrients and enzymes of either plant-based food or meat. If a person began to eat all of his food uncooked, would he lose weight? Yes. Can he permanently have an optimal weight and good health from this way of eating? No. If we never eat dairy foods with fruit, which is one food-combining principle, will we lose weight? Maybe. If we lost weight, would this be a permanent condition? No.

Here is a special category of fasting, whose effect is not primarily about calorie reduction, according to those who practice it:

-Intermittent fasting

The idea behind this practice is to contain whatever it is that we eat during the day within a narrow window of time. This is most easily done by

[8] Abu, Akua; Cooked Meat Provides More Energy; The Harvard Crimson November 9, 2011 "Harvard researchers have demonstrated for the first time that cooked meat provides substantially more energy than raw meat"

extending the overnight fast by several hours. It is usually described as a period of twelve or more hours. If someone woke up at 7 a.m., after an eight hour sleep, having eaten right before falling asleep, and he did not eat again until noon the next day, that would be a thirteen hour fast. However, most people do not eat the second before falling asleep, so the period of fasting, in this example, might actually be much longer. Did he eat at 11 p.m. and, then, quickly pass out? Likely not. Long before anyone was calling it intermittent fasting, people routinely practiced this when they avoided breakfast[9]. Even if they drank a cup of black coffee in the morning before dashing off to work, they still had not broken their fast. The inclusion of a little cream and/or sugar would barely qualify as having broken it. This practice is supposed to have multiple benefits for the body, from giving the digestion a rest, which is the claim for any kind of fasting, to avoiding damage to kidneys attributed to diabetes. Can anyone lose weight by

---

[9] Ofori-Asenso R., Owen A., Liew D.; Skipping Breakfast and the Risk of Cardiovascular Disease and Death: A Systematic Review of Prospective Cohort Studies in Primary Prevention Settings; Journal of Cardiovascular Development and Disease 2019 August 22; "Several studies have associated skipping (not having) breakfast with cardiometabolic risk factors such as obesity, high blood pressure,, unfavorable lipid profiles, diabetes, and metabolic syndrome......the pooled data suggested that people who regularly skipped breakfast were about 21% more likely.....to experience incident CVD or die from it than people who regularly consumed breakfast. Also, the risk of all-cause death was 32% higher..."

beginning to extend the overnight fast? Yes. Will this be a permanent effect and bring good health, to boot? No.

In the coming chapters, I will expound on the claims above and speak, first, about why the avoidance of calories cannot ever lead to permanent weight loss, no matter how many incarnations of it are invented.

Chapter 3

It Is All About The Calories

Multiple times every day I have heard references made about the evilness of calories. In a kitchen drawer, in the house where I grew up, there was a stack of type-written sheets of paper that intrigued me as a little kid. Each sheet contained the rules for a different diet. I wish I could remember what each one was all about. The only one I remember was one called the Gain Weight Diet. I was a skinny little kid, so I tried it. I don't think much, if anything, happened from following it. All the other diets in the stack were about how to lose weight using some kind of dietary restriction and calorie avoidance. So, from an early age, I was indoctrinated like everyone else where I live in the United States, to believe that we should limit calories in our diet. If we look for old advertisements from the 1950's, we can find some that promised women greater beauty by helping them gain weight with a pill. That desire to gain weight seems to have completely disappeared. What is ubiquitous, now, is the idea that calories are to be avoided so that weight loss can be achieved. "The fewer calories the better" seems to be the view of most. "You can never be too thin" was a phrase, popularized decades ago, which seems to have stuck. For many decades, this has been the case and it is my observation that the more this idea becomes widespread, the worse the "obesity epidemic" becomes. It started here, in the United States, and is spreading around the world. I hear the notion in television commercials, from wait staff in restaurants, from my friends, on boxes of food, on billboards, from proponents of the previously mentioned calorie-avoidant diets, in conversations I hear in my community and on YouTube. My doctor's office is also plastered with these messages. The findings from the weighing-in, first thing, when someone visits their doctor's office, often becomes the subject for a conversation about "eat less and exercise more" or, possibly, carbohydrate-avoidance, with the doctor.

When someone, archly, calls a food, usually dessert, "sinful", they are judging the calorie content of the food. When someone says, upon being offered "seconds" or dessert, that they "had better not", it is a judgment upon how many calories they have consumed already. When someone says they will not eat breakfast or lunch because they are going out to a party that evening, they say that in anticipation of the calories they will be consuming later, and they think they will be over-consuming calories if they eat earlier that day. When someone checks the label of a food or drink for the calorie content, it is because they think there is something inherently dangerous in a calorie. When I offer a friend half of my cheesecake, and they say, "I shouldn't", they are saying the calories will hurt them. When they will not eat breakfast, or lunch, or dinner, it is because they want to cut their calorie consumption for the day, (unless they say they are not hungry, which is another issue that I will discuss later). When a friend tells me she was "bad today", I know what will follow. She will then say that she ate too much. And "too much" has to do with calories. If my friend orders salad, when we are out for lunch, after slavering over the Monte Cristo sandwich with maple syrup dipping sauce on the menu, I know what that is about......calories. Skipping dessert? Calories. Drinking only water all day? Calories. "Diet" drinks? Calories. Waking up hungry, unable to get back to sleep, but refusing to get up and eat? Calories...(or maybe laziness, and believing what the magazines say about really "being thirsty" when she is clearly hungry, wide awake in bed in the dark). I am going on a bit about this, because I have heard it all. These are the things that I list when someone tells me that they eat too much. They argue that in no way do they need to eat more, but I think they do. In zero cases, when we have gone into the nitty-gritty of how much and how often someone eats, have I ever been convinced that they are eating enough calories. That is because I used to say and do those things, too. Later, I saw what really eating enough calories did for me, that was all positive. The disbelief comes because the calorie, as an enemy of normal weight, must be avoided at all cost in the collective mind.

I would agree that someone was eating enough calories if that person did not have any of the common ailments that affect our communities, in increasing numbers. I would agree with them if they had the energy to take control of their lives and live the way they want to live. I would agree if that person did not store fat with the slightest increase in caloric intake. Because these things are admitted to be true and because they are doing combinations of the previously discussed practices and diets, I know they are not consuming enough calories. Calories are energy. Never, ever do these folks believe that it is possible for their bodies not to put on excess fat if they eat as much as they want, of what they want, when they want it. As I have already said, but it bears repeating, we know that we are eating enough food to maintain good health when we cannot ever put on excess fat no matter how much we eat.

Calorie is the word we use for a unit of energy contained in food and used by our bodies when we move. That is not entirely accurate, however. Our bodies use calories even when we are not moving a muscle. In fact, most of our calories are used, on a daily basis, when we are not batting an eyelash. This fact is crucial to the information I am going to share. If I want to just brush the hair off of my face, I need more energy than I would if I did not do that. The number of calories we use each day, when we are lying perfectly still, is called Basal Metabolic Rate or BMR. This is how we use most of the calories we consume. This number of calories varies from person to person. We all need a certain number of calories while we are lying still. If we want to be healthy, with every organ and bodily process functioning as it should, we need to eat enough to ensure that we are. If we do not eat enough, we cannot maintain our body's correct operation. Especially while we sleep every night, our body tweaks all of our organs and other tissues to recover from any damage. Also, hormones and enzymes are made and utilized, and everything else that our body needs to be healthy is adjusted. If the energy is not there, the body has to prioritize more important operations and repairs. It simply must turn some things off in the hope that we will begin to take in more energy soon, and full functioning can resume. It prioritizes keeping the brain, heart and lungs operational, until even that becomes impossible. Some of the things that begin to suffer when we do not eat enough calories consistently, by which I mean daily, are skin, hair, nails, eyes, the thymus gland (which is part of our immune system), cognition,[10]energy, hormone production, reproduction in both sexes, normal menstruation, and so much more. If we want to move at all, the situation becomes much worse as movement requires more energy.

During the years before I understood just how many calories are really required to maintain good health, I was accidentally restricting my caloric intake by the practices of low-carb dieting and, for quite some time, the unnecessary elimination of gluten from my diet. I did not have celiac disease. Eventually, I was also practicing intermittent fasting and restricting my food intake to about 6 hours during the day. Here are the problems that began to appear in my body, after I began those practices. I had very deep grooves, pits, white spots and redness encircling the nail bed of my fingernails. Plus, they were very weak and split easily. My hair was getting thinner and losing its shine and after following a three week fast, it was

---

[10] Raichle, Gusnard; Proceedings of the National Academy of Sciences of the United States of America; July 29, 2002 Appraising the Brain's Energy Budget "Local changes in blood flow measured with PET during most cognitive tests are often 5% or less."

really coming out in clumps. The fast involved drinking fresh fruit and vegetable juices and eating dinners made up of salads, soups and lamb. So, it was not even a very extreme fast, but was, certainly, a sudden reduction in calories. During that time my throat over my thyroid began to hurt and I could not sing anymore. During the low-carb years, my eyes were weakening and I had to start wearing reading glasses. Plus, they felt dry and irritated. I got cellulite, for the first time in my life, even though I was losing weight. The weight loss, as it turns out, involved a lot of muscle loss, which became quite evident when I could not sit on a chair comfortably, at the table, without a cushion. My knees were so painful that many times, and for weeks, I would have to come down the stairs sideways, one step at a time, slowly. Sometimes, I felt so weak I could hardly climb the stairs. I bruised easily. The joints of my fingers were taking on that crooked appearance which occurs in osteo-arthritis from the build-up of collagen, which my body was using to shore up routine damage that could not be properly repaired. I had plaques in my carotid arteries. My iron levels were too low, in spite of the fact that I ate a lot of meat. My feet were becoming affected like my fingers. I had those little red blood spots called petechiae on my calves. My skin was flaccid and dry and I had developed a lot of those sun-damage brown spots called advanced glycosylation end products (AGEs). I had persistent rashes. I had a constantly stuffy nose. I frequently felt chilled. I had a bad case of rosacea, with general redness and spots that looked like pimples on my nose. My hormones were off. My digestion was bad. My blood sugar level was climbing. These things came on slowly over the course of years. I knew they were not normal and that there must be a solution, so I kept looking for clues in the scientific literature. My doctors could not help at all, except with drugs and ointments to mask the symptoms. Paradoxically, they were telling me to eat less and especially fewer carbohydrates, which were the very things that I had done, and was still doing, that had gotten me into the bad shape I was in. In fact, if there was a poster child for low carbohydrate eating, it was I. After years of trying, I had finally become perfect at sugar avoidance. I had been perfectly avoiding sugar for quite some time, when the doctors were telling me to eat lower carb. I was puzzled and frustrated.

Since I have addressed the energy shortage in my body by eating more calories, however, and given my body what it needs to repair everything, including a lot of carbohydrates, everything has been repaired. That includes any metabolic issues that were developing. I do not take any medications for anything and never have, except an aspirin or two in the early days of my recovery from starvation. Yes, I said starvation. It is starvation when the body is being consistently denied the energy that it needs to keep itself in good repair so that our organs do not atrophy and our body processes do not break down. Some starvation is so severe that it kills a person fairly rapidly. Some starvation is slow and relentless and takes years to kill us off, but it does kill us. I was starving and my body could not do repairs. I have had no surgeries and have taken no medicine, but when I stopped starving, everything fixed itself with the energy that was coming in.

Without doing any exercise, other than living my daily life, I rebuilt muscle and lost all of the cellulite. My flaccid skin tightened up and the brown spots began to fade and are still in the process of fading. My rosacea gradually resolved and my hair thickened up. My nails grew out stronger without any grooving, pitting or spotting. My intestines healed and digestion and elimination became normal. My thyroid began working properly, hormones normalized and my temperature came up to a consistent normal. I no longer have painful joints and my fingers have regained a straight appearance as my body has had the energy to perform normal healing of joint tissue. My sinuses are clear and I no longer snore. My energy is up for anything I want to do. The carotid artery plaques dissolved. There are many other things that have completely resolved and continue to stay in good repair. For example, a TMJ (temporo-mandibular joint syndrome) issue that I had for most of my life resolved itself in a three-day space of time and has never returned. I feel better than I have in decades. Without taking vitamins or supplements, I am completely well. I eat food. I eat anything I want, as much as I want to eat, and when I want to eat it. This is how the body is supposed to function and I know that even if a person has lived for decades, accumulating problems, it is possible for their body to return to a complete state of health.

I have also achieved a normal weight. It has been five years since I decided to start addressing my body's energy deficit. I began to lose weight 8 months after I began eating more. Because of a consistent high-calorie intake, my body has been remodeling itself. Let me explain what I mean. I previously stated, regarding all of the weight-loss methods that are recommended by someone and which so many people try, that a person can lose weight if they adopt any of them.....temporarily. Don't we all know, by now, that the effects of dieting are temporary? "Yo-yo" dieting is often spoken of as something that leads to more and more weight gain and a shift over time to an altered fat-mass to fat-free-mass ratio. I knew it was true for me, for a long time, but I did not know why. I do now. Even while I heard the warnings about cycling through diets, hope sprang eternal and I would try another one, hoping to achieve some kind of acceptable stability in my weight. Any change in our food intake or habits can result in weight loss, in the short term. If the effect is a reduction in caloric intake, or an adjustment in the source of the energy (like from primarily carbohydrates to primarily fat), any little shift can temporarily result in the body using its own tissue for energy. That tissue will be both fat and muscle. Because of addressing the energy deficit my body was suffering from, it has been allowed to return to a normal fat-mass to fat-free-mass ratio. That is what I mean by remodeling, as well as the return to health of all of my organs and tissues.

Metabolism is the rate at which a body uses the energy available to it. If a body is accustomed to a 2,100 calorie food intake, for example, it has adjusted its metabolic rate to cope with this energy availability. When it needs to, the body will use its own muscle and fat and even tissue from organs, like the thymus gland, to meet energy needs in excess of its usual rate of metabolism. Am I fighting an infection? The body needs more energy. Am I playing an unaccustomed game of tennis? I need more energy. Am I undergoing an unusually stressful situation? I need more energy. Is my kid learning to walk? I need more energy. Is my body healing a broken bone? It needs more energy. If I am healing from anything, like cancer[11], I require a great deal of energy. Obviously, our true energy needs will fluctuate over time, even daily.

Let's say that we eat 2,100 calories, like clock-work, every day. What happens when we start skipping breakfast? Our body suddenly does not have the amount of calories that it is used to having in a day. From where will it get the energy it needs to maintain the status quo? From its own tissue. It will use muscle, fat and organs. Weight is lost (the weight of the muscle, fat and organs that the body must use to make up for the lost calories). The needle on the scale is moving left or the digital number going down. The diet works..... until the plateau. "Plateau" is a word I became familiar with early on. My mom complained about it frequently. "I've hit a plateau", she would announce, at some point, after the initial happiness of

---

[11] Purcell S., Elliott S., Baracos V., Chu Q., Prado C.; Key Determinants of Energy Expenditure in Cancer and Implications for Clinical Practice; European Journal of Clinical Nutrition 8 June, 2016 "Despite their small size, tumors undergo high rates of glycolysis and lactate production regardless of their supply of oxygen....glucose turnover may contribute a great deal to high REE and muscle catabolism in cancer patients.....Estimations of additional energy expenditure associated with the tumor-bearing state ranged from 100 to 1400 kcal/day.....The energetic demand of a tumor, therefore, has the potential to substantially impact energy expenditure in certain patients."

weight loss. The "plateau" was when the weight-loss stopped. The above-mentioned hypothetical person eating 2,100 calories, who suddenly stops eating breakfast, will lose weight until the body makes the adjustments that it, absolutely, will make, to deal with this potentially dangerous situation. That is how the body sees what is happening. When the body has to dip into its own structure for necessary energy, that signals danger. If that person keeps skipping breakfast, the body will make adjustments to deal with the stress. Nothing is so stressful to the body as not having the energy it needs to run itself properly. Any adult eating 2,100 calories every day is eating too little and forcing the body to set priorities and lower the metabolic rate. It has turned down functions of organs like the thyroid and has been kicking the can of repair of other organs, joints, bones, eyes, muscle, etc., down the road, until there is the energy with which to do repairs, the need for which is mounting every day. The body has turned down the metabolic rate to achieve this sparing use of calories. The person, in our example, has less energy available to the system when they go from the already too low 2,100 calories to, let's say, 1,700 calories. The brain adjusts the metabolic rate downward so that the 1,700 calories the system now has available to it will be less quickly used up. This always means that something else the body needs to do will not be done. This is why dieters stop losing weight on the caloric amount that initially caused weight loss. This person, if they want to continue to lose weight, will have to up the ante and begin playing a game of tennis every day, to again force the body to use its own tissue, until the body figures out what is going on and again lowers the metabolic rate. Or, that person might start a low-carb diet, in addition to skipping breakfast, to force the body to again start using its own tissue for energy, until it knows it needs to make another adjustment to metabolism in an effort to prevent the body from quickly eating itself up. That is exactly what would happen if their brain did not protect them by lowering the rate at which they use calories by placing on the back burner a lot of things that need to be done. The more a person lowers their caloric intake, the more repairs and functions need to be tabled and the less well they will be. They become more and more damaged the longer this goes on. The "plateau" is the body's attempt to save its life, hoping for an end to the ever-intensifying "famine" it is experiencing. These kinds of increasing adjustments that a dieter has to make to continue weight loss, is what some call "tricking the body". We are the ones being tricked, by which I mean our intellects, if we think that it is possible to trick the body. The body always knows how to best cope with the decisions we are making, but those adjustments are not its optimal operation and in the long run we are not going to like the results. We will pay for it with increasing weight and illness.

It's obvious that trying to lose weight by decreasing calories is a negative, never-ending steep slope. When someone stops trying to starve himself {and his body will be vigorously trying to get him to eat more), he will put on fat. Why? Because fat is an endocrine organ[12]. That's right. It is not some useless bane of our existence. It is not even just a storage unit of energy against a future day. It has a greater purpose. It produces hormones. In a stressful situation, your body needs to produce more hormones to cope with the stress and, I repeat, nothing is more stressful for the body than too little food to operate itself. The body's ability to cope with all other stresses, physical and psychological, is enabled by enough energy. That is why the body, absolutely, will turn down the rate of metabolism at any sign that there is not enough food in the environment. So, we see what is going to happen if we have been on a new diet for a month and then decide to go to our friend's barbecue and treat ourselves by eating off of our diets? That's right. Our bodies consider the extra calories we consume at the barbecue a welcome relief. They use the extra calories we consume at the barbecue, calories above what our newly-lowered rates of metabolism have become accustomed to having, as a chance to grow our fat organs to cope with the

[12] Coelho, Oliveira, Fernandes; Biochemistry of Adipose Tissue: An Endocrine Organ; Archives of Medical Science, 2013 Apr. 20 "Adipose tissue is no longer considered to be an inert tissue that stores fat.....As an endocrine organ, adipose tissue is responsible for the synthesis and secretion of several hormones."

stress we have been under. Our bodies deliberately grow our fat organs to produce more hormones in the stressful situation of too few calories. Of course, doing that also ensures a possible supply of energy against the next day when there may, again, be the lack of food our bodies have come to expect. Of course, we feel guilty about breaking our diets at the barbecue, so we return to restriction the next day. The more this scenario repeats, the more fat is stored over time. We all know that this is the story from countless people who have been on a diet or many diets. They give up the diet and they weigh more, in the end, than they did before they began the last diet. When they keep repeating this pattern, in the eternal hope that they will eventually find the diet that they can live with forever, they become heavier and heavier[13].

What is ever offered as an alternative to "yo-yo" dieting? Constant calorie suppression is the method recommended in various guises. Even

---

[13] Chadt, Al-Hasani; 2020 June 26; Pfluger's Archiv; Glucose Transporters in Adipose Tissue, Liver and Skeletal Muscle in Metabolic Health and Disease "Adipose tissue represents a major endocrine organ that applies essential hormones and factors controlling whole-body metabolism, systemic insulin sensitivity, and energy homeostasis. Both the absence and excess of adipose tissue may lead to severe impairments of glucose homeostasis and diabetes."

those, who manage to, chronically, under-eat to the point that they always appear relatively slim, might be what is referred to as TOFI. That acronym stands for "thin on the outside, fat on the inside". The fat deposition and lean mass of this person has altered so that their limbs are thin looking but their torso carries excess fat. This visceral fat is stubbornly retained by the bodies of TOFI people to provide an emergency energy supply for the organs it is surrounding. TOFI people have a "normal" BMI and waist circumference, but the visceral fat is in there, not visible, like subcutaneous fat (fat under the skin) would be. If these folks are constantly under-eating, why does the body not just use the fat around the organs to supplement the body's caloric needs? Because, this is a stressful situation, with no end in sight, as far as the body is concerned. It is more sensible for the body to use its muscle, beginning with the largest muscle group, the gluteus maximus, for its energy needs, until that supply is as low as it can go. That is why, when I was thin, due to low-carb dieting and intermittent fasting, I had lost the muscle on my backside to the extent that sitting on an uncushioned chair hurt. After the gluteus maximus, the body uses the quadriceps, and so on. That is why the appearance of the buttocks and limbs is thin in TOFI people. Their body is not going to release the fat around the organs until things become very dire. Using the muscle also lowers the body's metabolic rate, a necessary thing to do when the body needs to use its own tissue for energy. As I said before, if the body did not lower the metabolic rate, the tissues would be used up too quickly and life could no longer be supported. This is the sort of adaptation the body is forced to make in a chronically deprived environment. Of course, the body will continue to use what tissue it can, for as long as the starvation continues. The adaptation where we store more and more fat occurs in a more intermittent style of deprivation, where we go on and off diets or just eat in a very erratic manner, from day to day. I once read a comment, by a doctor, who claimed that if a person ate even just two calories above her usual amount, those two calories would be stored as fat. At the time, I thought that sounded insane. Now I know that, yes, this is how it works for some people. But, not for everyone. Anyone who has been eating below the amount their body needs, even for a day, will indeed store any extra calories that are given it. Their body will grow the fat organ, as best it can, to save its life. The problem is, not that this person ate two extra calories, but that the person is never eating enough, consistently, to allow the body to stop storing excess fat[14]. To keep pushing the body to live on fewer calories is to

---

[14] Lifesciences.exeter.ac.uk Yo-yo Dieting Might Cause Extra Weight Gain 5 December 2016 "new research at the universities of Exeter and Bristol suggests...people who don't diet will learn that food supplies are reliable and they do not need to store so much fat...the model shows that if food supply is often restricted (as it is when dieting) an optimal animal-the one with the best chance of passing on its genes-should gain excess weight between food shortages...Surprisingly, our model predicts that the average weight gain for dieters will actually be greater than those who never diet."

push it toward death. What I did to get out of that situation was to stop starving it altogether. I started never eating below a baseline calorie amount that anyone my age, height and gender needs to eat. If I was in need of more calories than the baseline amount, due to increased activity or repairs my body was making, I ate as much as I wanted above that. When I did, my body grew the fat organ, in response to the deprivation it had been enduring, for the last time. It was saving my life.

If we are going to chronically under-eat, by eating 1,500 calories per day, for example, we will have to stay at that calorie amount forever, to not gain any weight, supposing that our body can lower metabolism enough to run on 1,500 calories. If we decide to start an exercise program while still maintaining that caloric intake, we will be making our bodies use even fewer calories for body operations because we are forcing it to use calories for moving itself. If we begin to eat more, in this scenario, we might make up for the deficit. If we provide even two extra calories, we will store them as fat. The body is not, yet, convinced that the famine is over and that more calories will be forthcoming. Until it is convinced, it is making marvelous adaptations to our internal environment to protect our life. We should appreciate this about any fat we have. The body has been saving our life, by growing the fat organ. In optimal nourishment circumstances, it would not have had to adopt this life-saving maneuver. That is why I say, emphatically, that we know we are giving ourselves enough calories when we do not gain weight no matter how much we eat. It is when we have been eating an amount of calories under what our body needs that the fat storage begins, with any calorie above the limited amount we have been eating. I was able to convince my body, over a long enough period of time (8 months, in my case), that the famine was over. I keep my caloric intake above what my body needs, at baseline, so that I never put on excess fat anymore. I am "fat-proof". However, if I became ill with a bacterial infection, injured, poverty-stricken or was in a real famine, I would store excess fat to make up for the stress when food was again available or desirable to me. That life-saving back-up mechanism is always there if we need it. The difference would be, that I now know to keep eating to get my body back to its normal metabolism.

The body knows what is an optimal amount of fat for each individual. Too many people disrespect their bodies. I want to, respectfully, use the illustration of dogs, because so many of us really love dogs and there is so much genetic potential for variation among dogs. Don't we love that variety? Chihuahuas and Irish Wolfhounds are both dogs, but what a difference! Can you love the physique of a St. Bernard as much as that of a Whippet? I do. Humans have quite a lot of genetic variability in their physiques, as well. There are quite a number of systems that have been developed that describe the variables seen in the human physique. There do seem to be some patterns. The ancient medical system of Ayurveda, for example, divides human physiques into three categories or combinations of those categories (called doshas). Those three correlate, more or less, to another system describing people as mesomorphs, endomorphs or ectomorphs. There are also a few systems where people, especially women, have been categorized as one of thirteen types or some other number. The one I have found most useful is the system developed by David Kibbe and described in his book Metamorphosis. There are many people who describe how to implement his system on YouTube. The reason I mention this, in this chapter, is so that right at the beginning we understand that healthy bodies do not all look the same. We may acknowledge that, but why do so many of us think that we can diet our way into looking like our favorite celebrities or our friends with the least fat percentage on their bodies? People do have different genetic body types, and the variations are many more than thirteen or any other number. There is more uniqueness to us, but it can be useful for us to know something about certain commonalities so that we do not think that physical traits that are common and perfectly normal are some singular problem that only we have.

What I like about David Kibbe's system is that he is not trying to "balance" everyone into some middle of the road ideal. He celebrates the individual. Rather than have everyone try to create an hourglass shape, his system is about enhancing the features that make a body unique and, in doing this, helping a person look more comfortable in their own skin. Nobody looks squeezed like a sausage into their clothes or in some other way awkward. One feature of the body that is taken into consideration is height. Another is the fat deposition, which varies among individuals who have a perfectly normal weight. Some people, genetically, have more taught flesh with less fat underlying the skin. Some are naturally fleshier, with more fat in cheeks, upper arms and thighs. In Kibbe's parlance, this is called "soft". All of these types are perfectly normal and will have these differences even while at a normal weight. All of these differences are beautiful. But, we have not been respecting this about ourselves. We think there is something wrong with us that we must remedy by denying ourselves what we need. We think we do not deserve to be treated with love and respect until we have altered our physiques in some way. We get ourselves into all of the trouble that we see the world is in, health-wise, by adopting this view of ourselves. This view is reinforced by society at large, for various reasons, which makes it difficult to break free of it. I think appreciation of the individual is the way to get us out of the psychological conditioning, as a society, that causes us to harm ourselves. We need to encourage young men and women to appreciate their uniqueness and the uniqueness of others so that they do not even take the first step toward harming their metabolism, by going on diets for weight-loss purposes. The road I traveled to recover from under-eating was a long one. It was not always pleasant. It is best not to have to do it, by avoiding the body-hatred that was its catalyst.

Let me describe how I got into trouble. I will bet many have done the same, to some degree. That skinny little kid that I was, when I was trying that Gain Weight Diet, turned into a curvier person at puberty. In Kibbe's system I am described as a "soft natural". This describes a person who is not narrow-framed, with width in the shoulders which are wider than the hips and with some softness of flesh in the upper arms and thighs. My curviness is mostly from the side view with a straighter appearance from the front. There is absolutely nothing wrong with this kind of frame and flesh. However, when I was sixteen, I did not appreciate it, at all. I envied girls I knew with other body types. I wanted longer bones and a narrower body, like some of my friends. I wished I had a flatter stomach and backside. More exaggerated shoulders compared to the width of my hips would have been nice, I thought. Those girls were more like the ones I saw in the fashion magazines I loved to read. I didn't really notice that some of my favorite actresses were more like me. I would have taken some comfort in that. After all, they were considered very attractive. I wanted to have that look that women who represent about 9% of the population naturally have and is the look that fashion models usually have, though. So, at some point I went on my first calorie-reduction diet. This took the form of skipping lunch most days, while I was in high school. I also tried to just limit sweets. I didn't really think of it as "being on a diet", because it didn't have a name. It wasn't Pritikin's or Atkin's or anything. But, in my head was this idea that I should eat less and limit sugar consumption to gain those really slender thighs that I wanted so much. The idea that I was enormous became really entrenched when I found myself in a store trying on some Levi's jeans, with one of those narrow-framed girls from school that I admired so much. She happened to be trying on jeans in the changing room next to mine. When I discovered that the size of jeans that I had taken into the changing room with me were too small, I felt embarrassed and my school mate asked if she could get me the next size up. I agreed and she brought me another pair. Those did not fit either, and when she was not looking, I sneaked out of the changing room and fled the store. Trying on bathing suits was another stressful activity that I wanted to avoid. I just did not appreciate how I looked, then, but when I look at photos from those days, it really makes me angry. There was nothing at all wrong with the way I looked. I was slim, so I feel angry that some confluence of ideas made me think I wasn't and caused so much trouble in my life. I dare say that if we all look back at our photos from the day before anyone suggested that we were fat, we would see that we were not carrying any excess fat. We were just normal-sized people with a particular body type that was not often represented in the pages of fashion magazines. Whether the magazines should represent their readership is a subject much debated. Maybe we would have been less inclined to consider ourselves as less-than, if they had. Nevertheless, many of us thought that there was something wrong with us that we could manipulate and improve. We did not know that we were setting off a cascade of metabolic and physiologic events by going on our first diet.

After I stopped skipping lunch and dessert, I gained weight and kept it on for a time. I now know that this is how my body responded to save my life in the aftermath of the terrible stress I had been putting it under by eating too little food every day. The calorie restriction ended when I graduated from high school and my family moved to another city. We couldn't move into our new house as soon as we had intended, due to some problem with the well. We were staying in a good hotel with a good restaurant, compliments of my dad's employer. I had three meals per day in that restaurant and had dessert after lunch and dinner. It wasn't long before my mom commented that I was packing on some pounds. I don't remember doing much about it; but eventually, as evidenced by photos from that time, I regained my normal slimness. This lasted for some time, according to photos, and even after the birth of my first child, I regained my slim physique, at least within two year's time. I never considered myself slim at the time, though. I always considered myself bigger than I should be. I now see that view was not at all true. It makes me mad because if I had realized I was just fine, it would have saved me a lot of trouble and anguish over the years. I would never have gone on that first diet or I would have stayed in those spaces where I had returned to a normal weight after the weight gain which follows the end of calorie restriction. I would have happily continued eating what I wanted. That is where everyone takes a wrong turn, the first diet. They continue on the wrong path by not staying off of a diet, once they break one. I now know why I would return to a normal weight after ending a diet, if I stayed off of it for long enough. I will explain this, in the next chapter, as I explain what I did to recover forever from diet cycles. What I did is the only way to permanently regain a normal weight and good health. It is none of those things in the list in the introduction. None of those things worked.

Chapter 4

If You Had Food You Ate It

Let me restate two points from chapter three. If someone is going to eat 1,500 calories per day, they have to keep it at that calorie amount forever in order not to gain any weight. If they do this, though, they will not be able to stay well. If a person has not restricted calories in any way, ever, they shouldn't start. They should just keep doing what they are doing, appreciate their body and eat as much as they want. If a person gains weight doing that, then they have been under-eating, perhaps subconsciously, or have been ill and haven't felt like eating. What can someone do, who has restricted calories, to get out of the fat-collecting adaptations their body has had to make because of what they, unwittingly, have been doing?

I am going to expound on some ideas I mentioned before. We are in one of two states if we have previously restricted calories, with a possible third state, though very rare:

1. Someone began their first diet and after the initial weight loss, they stopped losing weight, so they kept restricting calories more until they achieved a weight they were willing to live with. That person maintained the suppressed weight by sticking pretty rigidly to a plan. If they deviated from the plan at all, they started to gain a little weight, so they quickly went back to the plan. They might be, as a result, what others regard as normal weight, maybe even according to BMI charts, but their weight is truly suppressed[15]. Alternatively, that person might be overweight by the BMI charts, nevertheless, their weight is also suppressed. BMI is not a great measure of anyone's ideal weight. I remember a story about a professional American football player told by, I believe, Covert Bailey, in one of his books called Fit or Fat. This player was constantly being criticized by his coaches for being

---

[15] Schmerling, Robert H., MD: How Useful Is the Body Mass Index (BMI)? Harvard Health Publishing, June 22, 2020 "Research suggests that BMI alone frequently misclassifies metabolic health..."

overweight. When the player had his body fat measured, he had 6% body fat, even though the BMI chart said he was overweight. Don"t go by these sorts of standard measures. People are not standardized. If someone is maintaining a suppressed weight, by restricting their caloric intake, whatever their weight is, they are living with a suppressed metabolism. Their body is not doing things that it needs to do. It cannot afford to. There is too little energy coming into the system, chronically. They are or will be sick, in some way, eventually. Their body is attempting to live on the fuel they are taking in through the diet, but only with a suppressed metabolism. It has already used what tissue, in terms of fat and muscle that it is willing to use under the circumstances. The body may not be getting enough of the vitamins and minerals it needs because, of course, the fewer calories someone eats the less potential there is for nutrient intake of any kind. If someone eats little fat, their body may be struggling to utilize the fat-soluble vitamins. All of these factors put the consistently calorie-suppressing person in a very precarious position. They might be slim-looking. They might be TOFI. They are not in the robust state of health they should be in. This category includes those famously non-fat French women who gain weight when on vacation in the United States. If they were eating everything their bodies needed every day they would not gain weight no matter how much they ate elsewhere or at home.

2. The other very common state for people to be in, if they have previously restricted calories, is the state I mentioned before, caused by the proverbial "yo-yo" style of dieting. This is what I call inconsistent eating or intermittent eating. The "yo-yo" dieter begins and quickly ends diets with some space in between, when they are not restricting calories. What I will say about "yo-yo" dieters is, in my opinion, that they are not eating disordered. Why do I say that? Because the reason why they fairly quickly end a diet and allow some space of a few months before taking up another diet is that they can't stand the restriction of a diet. That is a healthy state of mind. They feel pressured by societal body expectations to take up a diet, but they cannot tolerate the restriction for long. The body is trying its best to get them to eat and finally they do because depriving themselves does not make them feel well. Contrast this with someone with an eating disorder. The person with an eating disorder feels better when they are restricting. The thought of eating freely disturbs them. Their body is suffering because of constant restriction of energy, but to redress the destructive energy deficit by eating more is something they will fight against. An eating disordered individual is in a high state of anxiety at just the thought of eating unrestrictedly. Mind you, those with eating disorders can be in any sized body. The emaciated poster child is just part of the story, and someone with an eating disorder will be at any point on the weight distribution curve. Someone may begin overweight and end emaciated or normal-looking in weight, but have an eating disorder at

every point on that journey. Every starving person, who stops starving, gains weight. I repeat, every starving person, who stops starving, gains weight. So, our yo-yo dieter famously gains weight at the end of her first diet and ends up with more extra fat on her frame than she had before she began her first diet. This happens because of the life saving maneuvers her body initiates in response to having to dip into its own tissue for energy. However, she starts to panic because of this misunderstood weight gain and begins another diet. She hopes that the new diet will be more tolerable than the last. She tells her friends, "It's not a diet. It's a life-style change". Maybe she sticks with this one for six months. But, again, her body is screaming for the nourishment it is missing and our exhausted dieter ends the diet one day in a spectacular display of body care. She does this because she is not eating disordered, because her body is demanding to be cared for and she stops telling it to shut-up. Because she has been starving and every starving person gains weight when the starvation ends, she puts on more weight than she gained after the last diet. If she keeps up this pattern for long enough, she becomes much larger than she was[16]. It is not the dieter's fault. It is not caused by a lack of self-control. The body of an under-eating

---

[16] Strohacker, Carpenter, McFarlin; Consequences of Weight Cycling: An Increase in Disease Risk? International Journal of Exercise Science, July 15, 2009: "within a year of weight loss, 16 out of 28 women regained weight and had a 19% increase in body weight and a 26% increase in percent fat mass."

person is determined to get them to address the starvation. They do not have a psychiatric issue that is enabling them to forever ignore their body's needs, until they die of it. However, they are still damaging their bodies by this repeat performance of calorie restriction. It is not calorie excess that is harming them, it is intermittent deprivation. Their bodies need consistency to end the negative cycle. The folks who do this are simply doing what their entire culture is telling them the solution is to their dissatisfaction with their bodies, that eventually becomes a real overweight problem. No, the whole thing didn't start out as a problem at all. It began as a lack of appreciation for what they had and the cultural demands that are not about the health and true beauty of the individual. Of course, these intermittent eaters are the ones who are vilified for their weight and told they are unhealthy, but those who are more consistent about their calorie restriction, however slim they might look, are more consistently denying themselves health-giving nutrition. Both of these categories of calorie-restrictors will suffer ill health. Those who become overweight will be the ones, though, who are made to feel like gluttons, even though they are nothing of the kind. Remember the doctor who said only two calories will be stored as fat if they are two more than the restricted calorie amount we were formerly eating? It would take very little food in excess of the amount we were eating before to cause fat to accumulate. What that doctor seems not to realize is that, if that person was not already restricting calories, fat storage would not be the effect. I have spoken to family members of obese individuals who swear that their obese relative eats very little. Some people can restrict their caloric intake to 800 calories per day and still gain weight if they exceed that amount. That is a dangerously low amount. I repeat, these folks who have accumulated fat are not gluttons. We have to keep in mind, of course, that a larger body requires more food to be healthy. Height and weight are factors in how many calories someone needs. Obese individuals are never eating enough to recover from the obesity and deprivations their body is suffering, unless that individual is actually in recovery from former under-eating (whether an eating disorder or not) and experiencing the weight-gain phase of recovery. That weight-gain will be their last.

3. Now, here's the third extremely rare scenario, which I alluded to at the beginning of this chapter. Why so rare? Because, the world thinks that the worse thing that can happen to a person is that they become overweight or obese. People are driven to almost any extreme to avoid weight-gain or to solve the already existing problem of excess fat. So, if a starving person always gains weight after the starvation ends, how can someone stop the weight gain when they start eating what their body wants and needs? They can't. That is unacceptable to most people, so they fear to even try or to go the distance on a full recovery from restriction. They continue the consistent restriction or the intermittent restriction to try to wrestle any

possibility of gaining more weight to the ground. They imagine that once let out of the bag, the weight gain will continue forever and ever. It won't, but they can't trust it. Trust in the basic rationale of our bodies is missing. Most people have been taught to think that their body is out to get them and that unless they intellectualize and make preemptive strikes and squash down its reasonable requests, they will be in big trouble. The third thing that can happen to people who have previously been restricting calories, is that they stop restricting calories and they recover. They start giving their body the food it is asking for. They never, ever restrict food intake again, as they were doing, by tinkering with their diet. They begin to take in all the energy, macronutrients and micronutrients their body needs to fix everything that has gone wrong. They continue to eat what their body is asking for every day, so that the body can repair what needs fixing every night, while they sleep. They do this every day for years and years. The body improves and gradually the deposition of fat normalizes and this person becomes "fat-proof". This person can eat any amount of food every day and not gain weight. They can do this because they are not ever eating below the body's energy needs. They can eat above what they ate yesterday, two calories or two-hundred and they will not store them as fat. This was the state that I had achieved a couple of times in my life, accidentally, without knowing how or why. I have now achieved it again, deliberately, and am determined that it will be permanent. I now understand how it works and I have proven to myself that the science I found, about how the body works to protect us from the effects of starvation through growing the fat organ, is true. I am living it. I am not going to begin another diet, ever, and create another energy deficit that my body will have to react to. This will be achievable if I am never unfortunate enough to experience real famine through climate troubles or poverty. If I do experience either of those situations, and am able to experience better times, I will understand what is happening when my body gains weight. Every starving person gains weight when the starvation ends.

Number three is the only way to a permanent normal weight and good health. The best thing that leads to the same result is to never restrict our calories at all. That is by far better than having to recover from under-eating. The reason is that under-eating always causes damage. There are things the body cannot do while energy availability is low. After a period of under-eating, the body must fix the things it was not able to keep in good repair. However, if we already have restricted, any weight that can be called normal is achievable only through the recovery described in number three. If we have never suppressed calories, ever, whether consciously or accidentally, we are at a normal weight. We all know an infection can make us lose our appetite and lose weight. If we keep this in mind, we will not panic when we gain weight again when we start feeling better. If we keep eating what our body is asking for, our weight will normalize. Who can tell us what our normal weight is? No one. We do not know. The BMI chart does not know. Our mother doesn't know. Our husband doesn't know. Neither does our doctor. Our doctor or someone else might be able to tell by looking at us that we are not carrying our body's ideal deposition of fat. Maybe. However, many under-eating people are told they "look so good" when their weight is anything but normal and their body is suffering the ill health of deprivation. No one can equate a number on a scale with what our individual healthiest weight would be. None of them will be unbiased by the cultural indoctrination we have all had, to think of health, weight and beauty in narrow, unnatural and unhealthy parameters. So, who does know how much an individual should weigh and what the fat deposition of that body should be? Their individual brain knows. Not their intellect, trained by the culture. The brain and central nervous system, untrammeled by limited energy availability, can bring the individual's body back to its natural state, which is the form that, according to genetic inheritance, the individual was meant to have. The amount we will weigh in our healthiest state will depend on such factors as bone density, length of bones, natural fat deposition (for example, how much breast tissue a woman is naturally supposed to have), the size and density of muscle, how much water a body is carrying at any given time, narrowness or width of bones, how big a head is, and so forth. Only our body knows what those factors will optimally amount to.

When we trust our body to return us to our natural healthy state of being, do we need to know what the number is that represents how gravity is acting upon the mass of our body? What would the possible use of knowing that number be? We will not be attempting to manipulate it in any way. To attempt to do that, for any reason, would put a person, once again, in one of the two previously mentioned precarious states of being, numbers 1 and 2. Okay, Okay, I can think of a couple of reasons to know our weight. One, because we are boxers and need to know our weight class. Two, we are flying a helicopter and need to know how much cargo we can carry aboard. Three, we are recovering from an eating disorder and our care team needs to know that we are gaining weight. There may be others, but none of these has ever come up in my life. However, in no way do we need to compare that number with anyone else's number. Someone else's number means nothing compared to our own.

The way of being that I am describing is how people used to be before they knew about calories and vitamins and the hundreds of little manipulations they could make to the diet, with the idea of controlling weight. For the most part, in the history of the world, in every place, food was something we ate with our family and friends, because we needed the energy it provided, because we enjoyed it, and because it was there. If it wasn't there, it was mightily unpleasant and we ate with gusto when food was again available. We would go to great lengths to get it, if we needed to. It, usually, appeared with daily regularity, prepared by someone dedicated to the task of providing it. It was recognized that children absolutely must have it regularly to grow and thrive, and parents were very aware of their responsibility to make sure their kids had enough of it. Most people did not think of food as something to deprive themselves of, when it was available. If someone was hungry, he ate. There was, usually, some set schedule of mealtimes. There were often set times for between-meal snacking, too. People turned up at those times, set for meals and snacks, and were concerned if they missed one. People ate consistently, on a daily basis, and so avoided the effects of inconsistent eating. In this way, they avoided excess fat. They would certainly be affected if the food supply was shaky. If there was consistently a lack of food, they would be affected by infectious diseases to a greater extent. Tuberculosis was an infectious disease that people succumbed to when they did not have an optimally functioning immune system due to under-nourishment[17]. The more people were in control of what they could consume on an individual basis, the healthier

---

[17] World Health Organization; Tuberculosis; 14 October 2021 "The risk of TB is also greater in persons suffering from other conditions that impair the immune system. People with undernutrition are 3 times more at risk. Globally in 2020, there were 1.9 million new TB cases that were attributable to undernutrition."

they were. They were able to listen to their body's individual demand for food and thus address all of the body's individual nutritional needs.

Before people were intellectualized by popular media about their bodies and made self-conscious about them, most people avoided excess fat by simply eating on a regular schedule every day. The main problem they would face would be a lack of food because of poverty or famine. Another possibility for deprivation was in the case of a religious zealot who felt that depriving the body made them more spiritual. That person might have felt that the scripture's injunctions against gluttony or "over eating" were referring to meeting the body's actual needs, so, they would "mortify the flesh". Gluttony and overeating, as spoken of in spiritual texts, must be understood in the context of the practices of all-day banqueting and what people would do to help themselves eat beyond their body's desire for what it needs for health. Far from being just the normal satisfaction of their body's needs, those practices had to do with an attitude of greed and more closely correlate to some modern day practices that I will mention later, like bulimia[18]. Of course, there have always been starving people, but what is

[18] Marchetti, Silvia; CNN Style 25 November 2020 "'They had bizarre culinary habits that don't sit well with modern etiquette, such as eating while lying down and vomiting between courses', Franchetti said. These practices helped keep the good times rolling. 'Given banquets were a status symbol and lasted for hours deep into the night, vomiting was a common practice needed to make room in the stomach for more food. The Romans

truly unique is a time when people do not eat enough, out of choice, because they believe that it is best for their health. The war that people are having with their own body's needs is new, for the most part introduced in the last few decades. What is an individual body's actual need for calories and how do we know?

---

were hedonists, pursuing life's pleasures', said Jori, who is also an author of several books on Rome's culinary culture."

Chapter 5

What Healthy People Do

If two people were both women who weighed 140 lbs. and were 5-feet-5-inches tall and they were both 25 years old, would their need for calories be the same? No. Here is why I say that. What if one woman was raising a toddler? What if one walked to work every day, five miles there and five miles back? What if one was fighting an infection[19]? What if one had

---

[19]Segerstrom, Suzanne, C; Stress, Energy, and the Immunity: an Ecological View; Curr. Dir. Psychol. Sci., 2007 "A 175-pound man would require more than 250 calories daily to maintain a fever of approximately 2° Fahrenheit.........other immune activities that require energy include producing proteins and generating new immune cells in order to fight infection."

been suppressing her metabolism by under-eating calories for a while? What if one was a construction worker and the other one sat at a desk at the library for several hours every day? What if one of them was caring for an aging grandmother? What if one of them gardened on the weekends and the other went hiking? What if one lived five flights up in an apartment building and the other lived in a ranch-style house? What if one walked to the end of the drive for the mail every day and the other just had to reach around the door-frame to reach the box hanging on the front porch? All of these variables would make a difference to an individual's caloric needs and the more often any particular activity is repeated or situation experienced the more profoundly it will be a factor in a person's energy needs. We can determine the Base Metabolic Rate of both of these individuals at some point in time, but it will not account for variables like the work of the immune system at any given point.

So, how can we figure out how much we, as individuals, really need to eat? Well, there has been research into this subject. Those especially interested in this question have been those who help starving people recover, whether it is those who work with people with eating disorders or victims of war, those who train athletes or those who feed people in refugee camps. Those who work with refugees have had a target of providing a

2,100 [20]calorie diet or a 2,400 calorie diet "to avoid having to supplement the diet further". Below 2,100 calories has been considered starvation by these organizations. The ubiquitous reference of a 2,000 calorie diet on fast food restaurant signs and on food labels is just a convenient number to calculate percentages of nutrients. It is not meant to imply that it is the amount anyone should be eating[21]. So, at least here we have a beginning figure. There has also been research into how much healthy people, who have never suppressed their calories, do eat every day. The fact that they have never suppressed caloric intake is very important because if anyone has limited their calories, they will have to eat more calories, to recover from the starvation, than they would have had to eat if they had never reduced their intake of calories. The fact that the people studied were healthy would inform us that their bodies were able to fully function on the amount that they were eating. Proponents of the Homeodynamic Recovery Method of eating disorder recovery have provided references for the amount of calories individuals have been discovered to be eating who are completely well and have not ever restricted their calories. In following their recommendation for my own age, height and gender, I fully recovered, as I

---

[20] wfp.org/wfp-food-basket "2,100 kcal are provided per person in a WFP ration."

[21] edinstitute.org/blog/2011/9/14/I-need-how-many-calories "2100 calories is not what any average adult needs to maintain her health, weight and wellbeing.....2500-3500 Calories A Day. Yes Really."

explained before. The thing I want to emphasize is that the numbers of calories that I am going to mention are a minimum calorie amount. These numbers will be a minimum, not a maximum number. We have all been brainwashed to avoid calories, so I say minimum and someone will imagine they read maximum. I am never again going to limit my calories by thinking of any maximum number, unless I want to be overweight and unwell. Following are the numbers from the above referenced sources.

If a woman is 25 years of age or older, based on the research, she needs to eat 2,500 calories or more every day. This will enable her to keep her body in good repair. This is a minimum amount she will need if she has never, ever restricted calories. If I am in this age range and am a woman and have never restricted calories, I am well and I am already eating around that amount.

Studies have shown that when asked to self-report their caloric intake for the day, all people tend to under report how much they eat. They do this for reasons of conforming to social norms. They imagine that it is normal to eat less than the amount they eat, whatever it is. People tend to under report by about 25%. So, if someone is saying they eat 2,000 calories per day, the actual amount is closer to 2,500 calories. If I have been on some kind of diet or have been exercising in an obsessive way, or both, I will have to eat considerably more than 2,500 calories daily to recover from the energy deficit I accrued and allow my body to return to its natural fat-mass-to-fat-free-mass ratio. I will either gain the amount of weight my body needs to gain, to become its normal self or, more likely, temporarily grow some excess fat organ then lose it again, to cope with the stress I have put it under, by starving it. This is exactly the reasoning I engaged in before I started allowing myself to eat more, much more, than that baseline 2,500 calories for my age, height and gender. What I deduced would happen is exactly what happened. After overshooting my previous weight by about 50 pounds over an 8 month period (during which I had gained weight then stabilized), my weight started coming down and has never stopped. The greatest weight loss happened over a period of a couple of years, which allowed my skin elasticity to also recover. Also, all through that period, I was feeling better physically in all of the ways I mentioned previously. For another couple of years smaller amounts of weight loss were still remodeling my physique. I am in my normal-sized body now, but fat is still being removed, at intervals, from my abdomen and the back of my arms. These are the last places from which the body will allow the fat organ to be removed. I had to learn to trust that my brain knows what is required where energy is concerned, and when it is a good idea to let go of the fat organ. This is not rapid weight loss, but it is permanent, and at no time did I have to deny my body the food it wanted, which are the two best things about the success I have had with this method of weight loss. I lost weight by always eating plenty of all the foods I want. Also, I never will gain weight again as long as I am making sure I never under-eat.

If the above woman, 25 years of age and older, is under 5 feet tall, she may cut the 2,500 calories by 200 calories per day, but there is little point in doing this, as it is a minimum calorie requirement to maintain a healthy body anyway. I will later explain why it does not matter if someone eats above 2,500 calories. Very important to realize is the fact that if people are carrying around an overgrown fat organ, to cope with the stress they have put their bodies under, they will definitely have to eat more than the 2,500 calories to recover and allow the body to eventually let go of the enlarged fat organ. Again, 2,500 calories is for a woman aged 25 and older who has never restricted calories. The reason for needing to eat more if we are carrying around excess fat is that fat is not biologically inert. Fat is biologically active. A larger body requires more calories, whether in terms of height or weight. The brain considers it very dangerous to let go of fat when there is not enough food coming into the system. Only when absolutely forced, to keep you alive, will it do this. But, under the stressful circumstances of any lack of calories, it will absolutely store what it can, when more food is available. We are losing ground when we do not provide the necessary calories.

What about 600 pound people we see on television, eating an enormous amount of food? Surely that proves that "morbid" obesity is caused by eating too much. No. It isn't proof of any such thing. Those folks started out doing that very first diet, like I did. They have dieted more than other people. They have been very, very inconsistent eaters. Each time they restricted calories their bodies compensated for the stress by growing the fat organ. Every time this happened, they tried another diet, with the result that they collected more fat, and had to grow more muscle to carry that amount of weight around, over time. To characterize them as people who never tried to lose weight and people who lack self-control is really wrong and unfair. They have gotten into the trouble they are in because they have tried so much of the bad advice out there. These folks need to eat the amount of food they are eating, because their bodies are bigger. They need to eat even more and more consistently, to ever lose the fat they have and be able to keep it off forever. It is a terrible mess, but they are victims, even more than the rest of us, of bad advice and a sick diet culture. Of course, it is ridiculous to think that these people have blithely been gaining more and more weight, to that extreme, without trying to do anything about it. Of course they have tried, given our culture's emphasis on thinness for social acceptability. Yes, you will see them during periods of non-restriction, but their restriction periods are not even going to look like anyone else's restriction because of the larger body's need for more calories. It is the restriction-non-restriction cycles that cause an enlargement of the fat organ. They must eat more now, due to their bigger size, to maintain body function. Also, don't try to tell me about the man who did not eat for a year and lost the enormous amount of fat he had. Yes, it's true. There was such a man, named Angus Barbieri, from Scotland. Of course, when someone forces their body, through absolute starvation, to use its fat organ to keep them alive for as long as possible, it is going to do it. A person with a larger fat organ is going to be able to live off of it for longer than a person with no enlarged fat organ. That does not mean that absolute starvation will not take a terrible toll on their body. It is amazing that he was able to survive the year, for various reasons of biology. However, he died early at age 51. I have read the statement that he died of "natural causes", meaning disease and not murder. It is not natural to die at age 51.

If someone is a man 25 years of age or older, who is over 5 feet 4 inches tall and has never restricted calories or is a woman under 25 years of age and is over 5 feet tall and has never restricted calories, they should eat 3,000 calories or more every day. All of the provisos and points about height and weight, in the above paragraphs, apply for them, as well. Another mitigating factor is activity level, This goes for all height, age and gender categories. If a person has a physically demanding job or exercises a lot they will need more calories on a daily basis than the baseline amounts given. If someone has a toddler, they have a physically demanding job. That proviso goes for the final category, as well.

If someone is a man under 25 years of age, and above 5 feet 4 inches tall, and he has never restricted calories, he should eat 3,500 calories or more every day. Notice, again, the phrase "never restricted calories". To reiterate, the fact of someone having ever gone on a diet or even having unconsciously restricted calories below these minimum amounts, will mean that he or she will have to eat more to make up for the energy deficit. Their body was putting off repair processes, down-regulating other processes and slowing the metabolism during the restriction. Their body now has to make up for lost time and energy. Therefore, it is baseless and futile to criticize someone for how much they eat, as if we know the amount they should be eating. No one has any idea what is going on inside an individual's body that is requiring them to take in the energy they are consuming. If it is the health of the body we care about, we want to see people nourishing themselves well with enough calories.

Now, while we are talking about calories, let me tell you about Billie Craig. I want to tell you about this man from the United Kingdom, because someone is surely thinking, "But, what if I eat some ridiculous amount of calories, like 6,000, for goodness sake! Surely I would get fat. I'm afraid that I would eat that amount if I let go of all the controls I am applying to my appetite every day". Billy Craig, at one time worked as a gym instructor. Even though he exercised every day, including every holiday, he still "wobbled" as he put it, by which he means that he still carried excess fat. Billy says he has Asperger's. This is what makes him, in his opinion, very fixed on meeting a goal, once he has set it. He has written about his 6,000-calorie, every day for a year, "no diet, diet" experiment on his own website. Without fail, he ate 6,000 calories every day and he lost weight to the point that he decided not to continue to eat that much because everyone was telling him he was too thin and needed to eat. Billy writes about why it works that way, biologically, as I do. And in case someone wants to say he ate super "healthy" or intermittent fasted or something, no he didn't. He ate on a regular schedule. This, in his opinion and mine, contributed to a pretty rapid weight loss. The body loves regularity. He ate at 2 a.m. every day, as well as at regular intervals throughout the daytime hours. He describes in an article for Matt Stone's 180 Degree Health website[22] what he ate. Anything easy to track the calories of, was what he

---

[22] Craig, Billy; 180 Degree Health Newsletter; Issue 4 March 2014; 6000 Calorie Weight Loss "I did it for one reason, and for one reason only--to prove to a bunch of female clients in a globogym that it was all about the pattern, the routine, and the message that you send to your body to say that food will arrive every day from now 'til forever."

ate, whole packets of bagels with cheese spreads, whole loaves of bread, and frozen dinners, etc. So, not what most people consider "healthy" and very rich in refined carbohydrates, and of course rich in energy, with that daily 6,000 calories. I now know why this large amount of caloric intake worked for Billy. Something like this worked for me. Billy embarked upon this experiment for the same reason that I did. He saw how the body really works and he wanted to prove to his clients at the gym that it was not eating too much that made them fat. It is quite the opposite. I wanted to stabilize myself at a normal weight and also prove that there is a reason that people get progressively heavier, which has an inverse relation to how much they are eating.

I did not eat 6,000 calories every day, but I ate as much as I could, keeping intake consistently above 2,500 calories. I had been severely under-eating as a low-carb dieter and "intermittent faster". I had been eliminating foods and groups of foods, one by one, as my intestines were increasingly damaged by lack of glucose and the calories that would have enabled repairs. I had eliminated cow's dairy products and gluten and was increasingly finding it difficult to feel good after eating any kind of food, at all. I had finally achieved a long-term goal of completely eliminating any added sugar sources. I had been eating perfectly sugar-free for a very long time. I was confused by my declining health and state of emotional well-being, because I was eating so perfectly "healthy", I thought. As someone who had been studying nutrition for so long, I had absorbed a lot of untruthful notions about food and was definitely "orthorexic[23]". I was overly concerned with the so-called "cleanness" of food. I needed to reacquaint myself with what a normal amount of food is. I started with the 2,500 calorie minimum as noted above for my age and height. That was surprisingly difficult to achieve, at first, for reasons that I will soon explain. Of course, because I had been restricting, I needed to eat above 2,500 calories to make up for the energy deficit I had accrued and heal damage. At the same time, I reintroduced sugar[24], gluten-containing foods and cow's dairy products[25] into my diet. Little by little, starting with a tablespoon of

---

[23] National Eating Disorders Association; Orthorexia: "Although not formally recognized in the Diagnostic and Statistical Manual, awareness about orthorexia is on the rise....means an obsession with proper or healthful eating,"

[24] Chadt, Al-Hasani; 2020 June 26; Pfluger's Archiv; Glucose Transporters in Adipose Tissue, Liver,, and Skeletal Muscle in Metabolic Health and Disease "Glucose represents the major source of energy for most tissues of the body."

[25] Forsgard, Richard A.; The American Journal of Clinical Nutrition, Volume 110, Issue 2, August 2019 Lactose Digestion in Humans: Intestinal Lactase Appears to Be Constitutive, Whereas the Colonic Microbiome is Adaptable "in lactase deficient individuals lactose feeding supports the growth of lactose-digesting bacteria in the colon, which enhances colonic lactose processing and possibly results in the reduction of intolerance symptoms. This process is referred to as colonic adaptation. In conclusion,

grass-fed yogurt, I moved to any yogurt in increasing amounts, then cream, then raw milk, then grass-fed from the grocer, then any kind of milk product at all. It worked beautifully. At first, I would have reactions to the milk products, but I persisted and can now have any food at all with no allergic reactions or digestive issues or malaise. My symptoms may or may not have been related to the lactose component of milk. It is possible that I was reacting to other constituents of milk, possibly a protein and not a sugar (like lactose). Nevertheless, it did take some adjusting. My body may have had to again start making some digestive enzymes that it had not needed to make when I gave up dairy or any of the other foods that I had eliminated. It took some time for my intestines[26] to heal, but, eating these

---

endogenous lactase expression does not depend on the presence of dietary lactose, but in susceptible individuals, dietary lactose might improve intolerance symptoms via colonic adaptation. For these individuals, lactose withdrawal results in the loss of colonic adaption, which might lower the threshold for intolerance symptoms if lactose is reintroduced into the diet."

[26] Yan H., Hjorth M., Winkeljann B., Dobryden I., Lieleg O., Crouzier T.; Glyco-Modication of Mucin Hydrogels to Investigate Their Immune Activity ACS Applied Materials and Interfaces 2020 April 17   "Mucins are a family of glycosylated proteins, and up to 80% of their mass is composed of O-glycans. Mucins are found bound to the cell membrane as part of the glycocalyx or secreted to form the mucus gel protecting the epithelium against irritants and pathogens and to provide hydration and lubrication."

foods again, and especially eating sugar sources[27], allowed my body to heal with the abundant energy that I was now supplying it. With the healing, my appetite came back and I was able to increase the amount of calories that I could eat. My body's metabolism was speeding up and needed more calories, so it demanded more, through increased hunger. I had to force myself, at first, to meet the 2,500 calorie minimum, but then it became easy to keep my eating above that amount to more quickly enable all the healing I needed to do and eventually lose the excess fat that had accumulated during the first 8 months of my recovery.

---

[27] Jaminet, Paul; Dangers of Zero Carb Diets, II: Mucus Deficiency and Gastrointestinal Cancers; Perfect Health Diet website, November 15, 2010 "If, for whatever reason, mucin production were halted for lack of glucose, we would have no tears, no saliva and no gastrointestinal or airway mucus...Fasting and low-carb ketogenic diets are therapeutic for various conditions. But, anyone on a fast or ketogenic diet should carefully monitor eyes and mouth for signs of decreased saliva or tear production. If there is a sign of dry eyes or dry mouth, the fast should be interrupted to eat some glucose/starch. Rice is a good source. The concern is not only cancer in 15 years; a healthy mucosal barrier is also essential to protect the gut and airways against pathogens."

Why did I have to force myself to eat enough, at first?[28] If someone is in a "fat-burning" metabolism, their body does not have enough fuel coming into the system from the outside environment, especially enough carbohydrates, to keep it from having to use its own tissue. The body can use fat for fuel, except for the brain, but this is not the preferred fuel source for most cells. This is a backup mechanism when glucose from carbohydrate[29] is not being supplied from the diet in adequate amounts. It is not supposed to be a long-term solution for the body. The body is forced

---

[28] Article: eatingdisordertherapyla.com; Seven Reasons You Should Eat When You're Not Hungry by drmuhiheim; April 30, 2019 "Just off the top of my head, I can think of a lot of reasons to eat when not hungry.....Regular meals are critical to getting all of your body functions to work properly again. One of the reasons you may not be feeling adequate hunger could be delayed gastric emptying, which occurs when someone is undereating and food remains in the stomach much longer than it should. One of the consequences is low appetite. The solution: eat regularly as prescribed, even if you're not hungry."

[29] Bilsborough SA, Crowe TC; Low Carbohydrate Diets: What Are The Potential Short-And Long-Term Health Implications: Asia Pac J Clin Nutr, 2003 12(4):396-404 "what potential exists for following this type of eating plan for longer periods of months to years. Complications such as heart arrhythmias, cardiac contractile function impairment, sudden death, osteoporosis, kidney damage, increased cancer risk, impairment of physical activity and lipid abnormalities can all be linked to long-term restriction of carbohydrates in the diet. The need to further explore and communicate the untoward side-effects of low-carbohydrate diets should be an important public health message from nutrition professionals."

to use its own tissue, especially the muscle tissue (which can provide a lot more necessary glucose to the system than fat can) to provide a constant supply of glucose to the brain cells and every other cell of the body[30]. The body cannot afford to not be at 100% of the fuel it needs, at all times, even at a reduced metabolic rate. There is only so far it can be turned down and we stay alive. So, it does the best it can with its own tissue availability and it does not constantly try to come up to 100% production from less, but rather provides a higher percentage of fuel for itself and clamps things down to 100% using hormones, like insulin. There is, in that case, glucose eliminated in the urine. So, if a body is using its own tissue for fuel, in a constant stream, it won't drive us to seek as much food for fuel. It will be necessary to introduce more food from the external environment into the internal

[30] Laugero K.D. A New Perspective on Glucocorticoid Feedback: Relation to Stress, Carbohydrate Feeding and Feeling Better; J. Neuroendocrinology 2001 September 13, "In this review, I discuss findings that have led us to view glucocorticoid feedback in the HPA axis in a new light Much of what has precipitated this view comes from a very surprising finding in our laboratory; sucrose ingestion normalizes feeding, energy balance and central corticotropin releasing factor expression in adrenalectomized (ADX) rats.....Taken together, recent findings of the well-known importance of glucocorticoids to feeding and energy balance, and the modulatory actions of carbohydrate ingestion on both basal and stress-induced activity in the HPA axis, strongly suggest that many metabolic (e.g. obesity) and psychological (e.g. depression) pathologies, which often present together and have been associated with stress and HPA dysregulation, might, in part, be understood in light of our new view of glucocorticoid feedback."

system, in an increased amount, to alert the body that the famine is over. Then the switch will be made back to the body's preferred mode of "glucose burning". It will take some time to convince the body that it is safe to make the switch. It is faster to make the switch from a glucose metabolism to a fat metabolism, because the fat "burning" metabolism is the back-up metabolism that is supposed to keep us from starving to death[31] when food, especially carbohydrates are not available for any reason. All it takes is about 12 hours of not taking in food to get the body to start using its own tissue. When we become entrenched in this metabolism, we will feel less

---

[31]Keys A, Brozek J, Henschel A; The Biology of Human Starvation: Volume I; 7.Physical Appearance and External Dimensions: "The clavicular outline in female inmates of an internment camp in southern France (Zimmer et al., 1944) was sharp and the hollow deepened. The padding of the shoulder girdle was greatly reduced, with a marked decrease in the breadth of the shoulders. The ribs became prominent, and there were the typical "winged" scapulae generally mentioned in field reports from regions in which undernutrition is prevalent (e.g. Adamson et al., 1945). The pectoral area was flat. The vertebral column stood out because of the reduction in the dorsal muscle mass. The waist was narrow, "pinched". The iliac crests became prominent. The wasting of soft tissues was particularly marked in the region of the buttocks, which became thin and flat with the skin tending to hang in folds. The arms and legs were spindly. The photographs, taken with the feet in standard orientation and at a constant distance apart, indicated a large increase in space between the thighs. Thus the diminution of soft tissues, including both the subcutaneous fat and the muscles , produced changes in physique characteristic of the "asthenic" body build. The bony framework remained the same, however."

and less hungry. I have been told by many people that they are never hungry and this is why. "Fat-burning mode" sounds good to people. They don't realize that their body is experiencing a state of emergency and in that state it is actually going to hang onto the fat on the body, if it can, because it is a precious hormone producing organ. That is why a diet "plateau" happens, as previously mentioned. The limbs and buttocks will lose muscle because the body would much rather use any expendable muscle tissue than fat. It will take carbohydrate eating to build it back. So, the limbs are scrawny, but "wobbly", as Billy Craig remarked, while the gut is sometimes distended or contains invisible visceral fat[32]. This is not the physique we were meant to have. Even if the waistline is a normal circumference, as In "TOFI" people, the fat is still in there, surrounding the organs, as previously mentioned.

There is another factor that makes it difficult to feel hungry enough to eat the minimum calorie amount after calorie restriction. It is that one of the things the body slows down, when it slows down the metabolism, is the rate of digestion, which affects the rate of peristalsis. By slowing down the

---

[32]Klitgaard, HB, Kilbak, JH, Nozawa, EA, Seidel, AV, Magkos, F; Physiological and Lifestyle Traits of Metabolic Dysfunction in the Absence of Obesity; Curr Diab Rep 2020 Mar 31   "Individuals with metabolically unhealthy normal weight (MUNW)......have a preferential accumulation of fat in the upper body (abdominal subcutaneous and visceral adipose tissues) and the liver, but not skeletal muscle"

rate of digestion, the body can not only extract more nutrition from what little the dieter is eating, but also use less energy, which is what a slow rate of metabolism is accomplishing. Someone with the condition called gastroparesis[33] is suffering from this effect of low caloric intake. I was suffering from that. So, yes, I did have to force myself to track the amount of calories I was eating, at first, to ensure that it was enough. My body was not used to utilizing calories from the external environment in sufficient amounts. By increasing my food intake, I increased my metabolism and my rate of digestion increased, as well. One underappreciated fact about regular bowel movements is that distending the stomach wall by eating enough food, in one sitting, to cause the effect of "feeling full", is what initiates the waves of muscle contraction that move things through the intestines[34]. Again, it didn't take any medicine to fix the gastro-paresis, in my case, just enough food to get things moving again.

---

[33] Rosen, Elissa MD; Gastroparesis, March 18, 2019; gaudianiclinic.com blog "In those who have restricted calories resulting in weight loss, whether in the setting of clinically evident eating disorder or even with relative energy deficiency in sport (RED-S), movement of food and waste through the gastrointestinal tract can be slowed....it is believed to be in part due to an attempt for the body to conserve energy during periods of low energy input. Delayed emptying of food from the stomach, also called gastroparesis, can lead to early fullness, bloating, abdominal distension and nausea."

[34] Kajal, Thavamani; Physiology, Peristalsis; StatPearls [Internet] March 1, 2021 "The stretching of the gut stimulates peristalsis."

The only useful time to count calories is when someone has lost touch with what enough food is. They do not feel hungry because of fat "burning" and gastroparesis so they cannot, at first, rely on their body to tell them how much they need to eat. If we need to count calories, it is only so that we can ensure we are eating enough of them, not to restrict them. We can free ourselves of the concern over calories quickly if we are completely onboard with eating enough to re-nourish ourselves. If someone relapses into restricting mode, they need to return to paying attention to calories, temporarily, to get back to the amount of calorie consumption they need to stay healthy.

So, am I talking about Intuitive Eating, with capital letters? No, I am talking about listening to my body only when I have returned to some state of normal metabolism, so that I can trust it. The way the phrase "Intuitive Eating" is being currently used is as another kind of diet to follow, with rules. If there are rules, it is not intuition. The healthy body, of a person who has never restricted food, does know what it needs to eat, how much and when, but it is easy to get into bad habits by intellectualizing food intake. If we start denying the body because of work hours and other demands, placating other people as to when we eat, so as to eat with them according to their irregular habits, or suffer an illness which affects our appetite or just decide that cutting calories will give us the body we want, then we can easily get into trouble. We do have to listen to what our individual body is telling us as to what we need. Culture and demands of life will sometimes interfere with being able to do this, so the above calorie guidelines are offered, as minimum amounts. It is not going to hurt a person, at all, to eat above those amounts, to whatever extent he feels the need. That is how he is going to get well from the cumulative damage that has happened to his body by chronically or intermittently denying it the necessary calories, for however long he has been doing that. The actual amount of calories someone's body will need will naturally vary from day to day. One day, because of that jog she went on, she will eat more. If her niece, age three, spent the day at her house, she'll need more to eat. If a cold is coming on, she'll need more fuel to fight the infection. In fact, research has shown that when we are fighting a viral infection, we will usually desire to eat more glucose than we will if we are fighting a bacterial infection. It can be dangerous to force someone to eat when their body is trying to kill off bacteria[35]. The body is trying to starve the bacteria. The expression "feed a

---

[35] Wang A, Huen SC, Luan HH. Shuang Yu, Zhang C. Gailezot JD, Booth CJ, Medzhitov R: Opposing Effects of Fasting Metabolism on Tissue Tolerance in Bacterial and Viral Inflammation; Cell, vol. 166, issue 6, 8 Sept. 2016, pages 1512-1525. "Here we report that, whereas nutritional supplementation increased mortality in Listeria monocytogenes infection, it protected against lethality of influenza virus infection. The causative component of food was determined to be glucose, and this effect was

cold, starve a fever" may reflect some instinctive knowledge of what was going on with different types of illness. No exact number can be determined that each individual will need on a daily basis except to say that a healthy body needs, at least, such and such number of calories. I know that if I feel like eating 3,000 or 3,500 calories one day, it is not going to hurt me, in any way, or make me fat. I have eaten that and more many times, since embarking on re-nourishing my body, and it has never resulted in anything but weight loss for over four years. I have only become slimmer and more and more well by ensuring that I eat everything I want in the amount I want, when I want it. I listen to what my body wants because I've learned that my central nervous system interacts with the outside world for just this purpose, to tell me what my body needs. It will indicate to me, according to

---

largely independent of inflammation or pathogen burden. To study the differential effects of glucose metabolism in bacterial and viral infection and sepsis generally, we utilized lipopolysaccharide (LPS) and poly (I:C) models of sepsis and found that, whereas therapeutic blockade of glucose utilization with 2-deoxy-D-glucose (2DG) protected against LPS-mediated sepsis, it was uniformly lethal with poly (I:C) sepsis. We found that, whereas glucose was necessary for adaptation to and survival from the stress of anti-viral inflammation by preventing initiation of endoplasmic reticulum (ER) stress-mediated apoptotic pathways, glucose prevented adaptation to the stress of bacterial inflammation by inhibiting ketogenesis, which was necessary for limiting reactive oxygen species (ROS) induced by anti-bacterial inflammation. Our study elucidates how specific metabolic programs are coupled to different types of inflammation to regulatge tolerance to inflammatory damage."

the things available in my environment, that it wants one thing for one nutrient need or amount of calories over another thing. On another day, it will want the thing that was not at all appealing to it before. I am talking about listening to craving and hunger, because that is how we know what our bodies need. A big problem is when there is not, in the external environment, what bodies need to be healthy. World War II was a time when many were suffering from that problem. An experiment was done to find out how to cope with the problem of starvation. The next chapter will explain.

Chapter 6

The Minnesota Starvation Experiment

The Minnesota Starvation Experiment[36] is integral to understanding

---

[36] Dulloo, Abdul G.; Physiology of Weight Regain: Lessons From the Classic Minnesota Starvation Experiment on Human Body Composition Regulation; Obesity Reviews 5 February 2021 "The publication of the detailed results of the MSE did not appear until 1950, that is, 5 years after the end of World War II. However, preliminary results about the efficacy of the various rehabilitation diets during the restricted refeeding phase were released earlier, with emphasis, to quote: "In relief feeding, calories are of overwhelming importance" and "unless calories are abundant, then extra proteins, vitamins and minerals are of little value". These bold statements, which were in contradiction with long-standing beliefs, were echoed three decades later when John Waterlow. who led most of the efforts focused on protein malnutrition, admitted that the hotly disputed "protein gap" underlying malnutrition did not exist and that people in developing countries only needed sufficient energy intake. These early challenges to the belief that excess protein intake would promote lean tissue growth and muscle function have since been reinforced by studies reporting that dietary protein supplementation did not improve lean tissue recovery during nutritional rehabilitation of patients with anorexia nervosa or in patients with protein-energy malnutrition and did not counter muscle disuse atrophy in young and older men. Furthermore, there remains today considerable uncertainty about whether an early and aggressive administration of protein and amino acids to very low birth weight infants is safe and efficacious.....the MSE has been the most influential scientific documentation detailing how starvation dramatically alters human personality, social eating behaviors, and basic body functions. It has been a guide in many aspects of public health and clinical medicine....improving famine and refugee relief programs of international agencies in the post war era of the United Nations......for exploring the impact of food deprivation on the cognitive and social functioning of those with eating disorders such as anorexia nervosa and bulimia nervosa.....for gaining insights into the clinical management of cachexia and weight changes related to illness and injuries and for underscoring the "famine reactions" of

what is known about under-eating. This study, embarked upon in the final months of World War II, performed at the University of Minnesota under noted physiologist Ancel Keys, has been the source that continues to inform the world about how to help at-risk populations recover from under-eating, since the latter half of the 1940's. The object of this experiment, begun in 1944, was to find out what it would take to return the populations of Europe affected by World War II, to health. They were starving and no one knew what it would take to help them recover.

Thirty-six young, healthy men were recruited to take part in the experiment. They lived and ate together for a year, at the University of Minnesota. Ancel Keys and his team took meticulous data during that time about how these young men were affected by semi-starvation. At first, the men were put on a diet of about 3,200 calories to stabilize them all in the same general playing field. They were supposed to maintain a stable weight, but some lost weight eating 3,000 calories, because it was less than they had been eating before they entered the experiment. Remember, our

---

compensatory hyperphagia and metabolic adaptations that might undermine obesity therapy......there is a large interindividual variability in the composition of weight regain and often a disproportionately faster recovery of fat mass than lean mass; this latter phenomenon, which has been coined as "preferential catch-up fat", has been reported in rehabilitated adults, as well as in children and infants showing catch-up growth...."

last chapter informed us that men who are healthy, who are under the age of 25, have been found by studies to eat around 3,500 calories every day, even if they report eating 3,000. The young men participating in the experiment, who were losing weight eating 3,000 calories, had to be given more calories to stabilize their weight. All of these young men had been examined before the study and were found to be healthy and of normal weight. This phase of the experiment went on for three months.

After three months, they were all put on an average of 1,570 calories from the kinds of foods available to the masses in Europe at the time, like bread, potatoes, and root vegetables. The goal was for them to lose 25% of whatever their body weight was before they started this six month phase of the experiment, the semi-starvation phase. Some, who were losing weight too quickly, were given an extra slice of bread or an extra potato to prevent a more rapid decline, but as the weeks went on, photos reveal that they all began to look like victims of the concentration camps. Mind you, this was on an amount of calories more than many diets recommend for weight loss. Keep in mind that the experiment was under controlled conditions. They were fed that calorie amount daily, consistently or slightly adjusted to control the rapidity of the weight loss, and they were not allowed to respond to their hunger by eating anything else. The absolute consistency, of this low calorie range, did not give the body any extra calories to store and allowed for the steady weight loss they experienced. Also, the experimenters did not allow the subject's metabolic rates to drop as much as their bodies would naturally have wanted them to. They were required to engage in educational studies, walk 22 miles per week and work 15 hours per week in the lab. These activities demanded more calories than would have been needed for just lying around. During this part of the experiment, the men's physical and mental condition deteriorated notably. This kind of experiment would not be considered ethical today. In 1944, those men, who were conscientious objectors from the war, were eager to do some kind of alternative service and were proud of their role in this vital information gathering. The men really suffered, however.

One participant broke the limited food requirement and was released from the study, so the buddy system was instituted for their walks and movie-going and so forth. This helped the men to deal with their quickly increasing weakness, as they couldn't even open a door alone. Other effects became increasingly noticeable. The men wrote about these things in the daily journals they were expected to keep, and the men who were still alive 60 years later, 19 in all, spoke of them when they were interviewed. For example, every little thing started to bother them, even their best friend's idiosyncrasies. I will here list most of the psychological and physical effects the men were experiencing during the 1,570 average-calorie-phase of the experiment. I observe, in great and increasing numbers, in the general population, all of these effects of their starvation. I live in the United States, and during my lifetime I have seen these things become more common here.

1. decreased tolerance for cold temperatures
2. unexplained dizziness
3. extreme tiredness
4. muscle soreness
5. hair loss
6. reduced coordination
7. tinnitus (ringing in the ears)
8. chronic lack of energy (manifesting itself in shuffling along, memorizing where every elevator was and looking for driveways to access the sidewalk, instead of stepping over the curb of the street)
9. chronic lack of motivation
10. obsessive interest in food (the subjects of the experiment developed an interest in reading and collecting cookbooks; one subject said that food became the one and only interest in their lives. These days, it might take the form of watching cooking shows, but not cooking)
11. eating rituals to make a small amount of food last longer
12. all interest in dating lost

13. irrational thoughts (one subject remembered seeing a boy traveling fast on his bicycle and feeling certain that the boy was going home to dinner and, for a moment, he hated that boy and felt guilty about feeling that way)

14. edema-swollen legs, ankles and faces.

15. anemia

16. neurological deficits

17. skin changes

18. negative effects on mental attitude and personality (Dr. Keys said that democracy and nation-building would not be possible in a population that did not have access to sufficient food); that means people just can't get along

19. lack of sense of humor

20. visits to psychiatric ward (by two participants who were later excused from the experiment)

21. habitual gum chewing

Extreme loss of weight was, of course, a necessary part of this experiment. The research team wanted to recreate the exact conditions that were being experienced by millions affected by the war. The point was to see what it would take to rehabilitate them. The effect being created was that of real deprivation of food. The men were being held firmly to the caloric intake they were allowed, by the parameters of the experiment, during the semi-starvation phase. They had lost 25% of their pre-semi-starvation weight and also 40% of their muscle mass. That was, as a reminder, on a 1,570 calorie per day diet, for 6 months. What happened next? The rehabilitation phase followed. The research team, at first, tried varying calorie amounts above what the men had been eating during the semi-starvation phase. They did this with the men divided into groups. However, they found that nothing worked if abundant calories were not given to a formerly starving person. They said that extra protein, vitamins and minerals were of little benefit unless something in excess of 4,000 calories was provided on a daily basis for some months. The researchers soon realized that ad libitum eating was the only way for the men to begin to recover. They stopped controlling their calorie amounts. Some of the young men were surprised that the rehabilitation phase was harder than any other part of the experiment. They lost additional weight, in the beginning, after they were given more food. This no longer surprises me. When eating-disordered people are being rehabilitated in a hospital, this has become a known effect of eating more. The extra calories (above what little they were previously eating) speed up the metabolism and so calories are more quickly utilized by the body. Hospitals know they must keep increasing the calorie amount they are providing in the early phases of recovery to keep up and not allow the patient to, dangerously, lose more weight[37].

The men said that lack of sex drive, tiredness and weakness were slow to improve. After the three-month rehabilitation period, they did not feel back to normal. Filling up their stomachs did not satisfy their hunger. Some felt more depressed than they had during the starvation phase, especially those who were, at first, in the group being provided the fewest recovery calories. We should not be surprised, by now, to learn that the men put on extra fat during the rehabilitation phase. Every starving person, who stops starving, puts on weight. This was weight that was above what they weighed before they entered the experiment. Also, remember, the men had

---

[37] Marzola E, Nasser J, Hashim S, Shih P, Kaye W; Nutritional Rehabilitation in Anorexia Nervosa: Review of the Literature and Implications For Treatment; BMC Psychiatry 2013 November 7; "Unfortunately, AN patients most likely will not continue to gain weight only by adhering to the recommended formula: 30/kcal/kg/day maintenance + 500 kcal/day for weight gain. Rather, we have found that the maintenance amount of calories needs to be increased at intervals to continue weight gain. That is, to continue gaining 0.5 kg per week it may be necessary - according to our experience - to do a step-wise increase of 10 kcal/kg/day every 5 to 7 days if there are plateaus in gaining weight. Some individuals with AN may require even more energy to achieve weight restoration and thus need up to 70 to 100 kcal/kg/day. So this may mean consuming 4,000 to 5,000 or more calories per day."

lost 25% of their pre-semi-starvation phase weight, but 40% of their muscle. Fat was faster to come back than muscle, so their body composition was changed, for a time. The men needed more calories after they had been starving than they would have needed if they had never participated in the starvation experiment. As Dr. Keys said, "Enough food must be supplied to allow tissues destroyed during starvation to be rebuilt". This repair work requires extra energy. Estimates of how long recovery took were from 2 months (for some) to 2 years (for others). All of the men felt that they had completely recovered at some point, though one of the subjects felt that the tuberculosis he developed after the experiment was related to the starvation he endured. Starving people are far more susceptible to tuberculosis.

Various phases of my rehabilitation and what I went through during my starvation years closely align with what happened to these young men. I would say that the differences are, in the length of recovery and that during my restricting years, which were longer than six months, I was, at least some of the time, eating calories in excess of a baseline amount. I was not under strictly monitored conditions and the famine was not real. I lost weight sometimes and gained it, in excess of my previous weight, over and over. If I had really been monitoring my caloric intake strictly or been in a real state of deprivation, as the populace of Europe had been in during

World War II, I would have been emaciated just as those participants of the experiment had been and the European population was, at that time. On the subject of starving Europe, during World War II, I want to address a common misconception about rationing of food in Britain. I have read many comments, guessing why people in Britain during World War II were healthier and not overweight. Most assume that they were eating fewer calories. Gardens were encouraged during the war and this would have supplied the highest possible nutrient content of fruits and vegetables, which were never rationed anyway. Every man, woman and child was given a ration book with coupons, beginning in 1940[38]. The rations provided about 3,000 calories per day, per person[39]. A family's caloric intake would have averaged out, with healthy men eating more and healthy women eating less and small children eating what they needed. The rest of much of Europe did not have this same regular caloric availability. The cited chart shows what

---

[38] iwm.org.uk/history/what-you-need-to-know-about-rationing-in-the-second-world-war "Every man, woman and child was given a ration book with coupons."

[39] bbc.co.uk/teach/rationing-could-the-ww2-diet-make-you-healthier "Throughout the war each person was allocated a scientifically devised weekly provision of specific foods...the daily calorific value was around 3,000 calories...Some manual labourers, such as miners and land girls, received extra rations."

was available to adults only, during various war years, with no averaging in of children's consumption to lower the average[40]. These are amounts of calories like the men in the Minnesota Starvation Experiment were given during the semi-starvation phase. It is the consistent caloric availability of guaranteed rations and the continued availability of fresh fruit and vegetables, along with the nutrients from the rationed commodities that resulted in a healthy populace in Britain.

I completely understand the feelings of the subjects that recovery was harder than the starvation phase of the experiment. It was true for me, too. When tissues are being destroyed and bodily functions curtailed because of lack of energy, it is a gradual thing most of the time. The damage accumulates over years, except in extreme cases of drastic and consistent under-eating. Eventually, we will notice that something is not working like it used to. Maybe, for example, we notice that our knees are cracking and there may sometimes be pain when we go down a set of stairs. What has happened is that over an extended period of time, the body has had to put off repair of the cartilage of joint tissue due to lack of

---

[40] history.ox.ac.uk/rationing-in-britain-during-world-war-ii "The table...shows daily consumption of calories and protein per person in the UK....Daily rations (kcal) average adult consumers in nine European countries."

energy to properly keep it in good repair. It is normal in the course of daily life to cause the oft-mentioned "wear and tear" to our cartilage. It is also normal for a well-nourished body to do repairs to that tissue with the abundant energy we provide it. If there is a lack of energy, however, the body must put off relatively unnecessary repairs in favor of keeping our heart, lungs and brain operational. The damage that occurs over time does not feel like much, in my experience, until the damage becomes so serious that it affects the operation of the joint in a big way. The damage seen in spines to bone and cartilage is another injury that can occur in those without enough energy to keep it consistently in good repair. The "wear and tear" theory is not accounting for the repairs that every well-nourished body will make to every bodily tissue. "Well-nourished" is a phrase often euphemistically used to indicate an overweight or obese individual. I hope, by now, that we understand that bodies carrying around excess fat are not those of truly well-nourished individuals. The excess fat is an indication of someone who is only intermittently eating enough during any given day. Another possibility is that it is the body of someone who is finally nourishing themselves properly and has gained excess weight for the last time. So, the euphemistically "well-nourished" person may be perceived as having damage to their knee-cartilage, as a result of carrying too much weight, but that is not what has happened. Truly well-nourished bodies heal.

Both, the excess weight and the unrepaired damage to knees, are symptoms of not being consistently well-nourished.

What feels like something is when the body tries to heal the damaged tissue. The body will constantly be trying to heal the tissue when there is any extra energy coming in. Most people do not live with consistent deprivation, but rather with intermittent deprivation. These are the people, like me, who become overweight and obese as they give up diets and take them up again. These are also the ones who develop joint pain, supposedly as a result of too much weight on their joints. What was really happening to me was the pain of healing, when a repair job had been put on the back burner for a long time, as a result of too little energy to do the repairs. Repair of all body tissue is a normal part of the life of every body. Repairs should be happening when they are small. With the intermittent energy availability in the case of a yo-yo dieter, the body initiates healing of the worn-away cartilage to provide the necessary cushion between the bones of the knee, in our example, or the spine or whatever. Healing is the thing that is painful, as it involves swelling and often itching, too. My body was moving necessary elements into the area being healed and it used water to do that. When my knees were being healed from their accumulated damage, they were swollen and painful. They had often been swollen and painful before, but that would come and go. I realized that the intermittent pain and swelling was caused by the times when I had given up the suppression of my caloric intake and my body had finally had the energy to do some healing. Paradoxically, the times when I did not experience any pain was when I was suppressing my calories and especially calories from carbohydrates. Of course, the damage was becoming worse as I was not providing my body with the energy to press on and complete the healing. If I had kept taking pain medication, like aspirin, the healing would have slowed or stopped. Sometimes, taking a couple of aspirin was useful to cope, but I tried to let healing happen without suppression of inflammation, as much as possible. When I gave up suppressing my calories forever, my body healed all of the accumulated damage and continues to do the small repairs which are normal for a healthy body. When the repairs are small and continuous, the damage stays small and the repairs far less bothersome, if we notice them at all. I never have painful knees anymore. If I damaged them, however, by slipping on ice, as an example, I would expect any necessary healing to involve some pain and swelling for a time. I would be wise to provide my healing knees with some extra energy to completely resolve the repair, as quickly as possible.

Our bodies are supposed to keep an ongoing repair job of everything that needs fixing every night, while we sleep and are not bothered by it. However, if the repairs are big, as they will be eventually if we are not supplying consistently large amounts of calories to our bodies, we will definitely be bothered by the repairs. That is why I found the recovery of health harder and more painful than any of the degeneration that had preceded it. What made it all worthwhile was that the inflammation, edema and pain that I experienced when something was healing was experienced for the last time. If I cut myself or break a bone, in future, I expect that swelling, pain and itching will accompany the healing. I finally understand what it all means and that helps me be patient with it and let the healing happen. If I had done damage to my lungs, so serious that I experienced a lot of edema in that organ, I would have had to consult a doctor to help me through that healing process. That would have been tricky, as taking anti-inflammatories stops or slows, greatly, the healing process. It would have required a nuanced approach of monitoring by a good doctor. I have become aware that healing is not a straightforward matter of feeling better and better every day. It is a very squiggly line upward, downward and all over the place. That is because less than ideal patches have been put on damage in the body, to use a metaphor. Those "patches" have to be ripped off and real healing must take place. The body knows how to incrementally go through all of the layers, but it takes time and some things can temporarily feel worse. Also, no two people are going to have the same experience during re-nourishment, because the life and damage have not been the same. Someone else's experience will only be so informative to the journey of another person. I now feel on a refreshing plateau of post-healing. Inflammation was a necessary part of my healing. What inflammation is not supposed to be is chronic. It becomes chronic when the organism has become so damaged that it is constantly trying to initiate periods of healing that never become resolved because the amount of energy coming in is never consistent. When I provided my body with consistent, abundant energy through my food intake, I stopped having chronic inflammation. Healing is no picnic, as the men in the Minnesota Starvation Experiment found out, but the only way out of the damage is through the healing process.

What do we learn, as take-aways, from the Minnesota Starvation Experiment?

1. If someone under-eats calories, even to a level recommended by many weight-loss diets, they will suffer tissue damage.

2. If someone under-eats calories, even for just six months, they will suffer psychiatric, neurological and personality damage.

3. If someone under-eats calories consistently, their body will eat up its own tissue for energy, and they will become emaciated.

4. If a person stops under-eating, he will gain excess fat and only lose it again by feeding himself enough calories, consistently, so that his body will feel it is safe to reduce the fat organ again.

5. If a person wants to completely recover from the damage done by under-eating, she will have to eat far more calories than she would have eaten if she had never restricted her calories.

6. Eating extra protein and taking vitamin and mineral supplements will not help someone recover if they do not consume enough energy for recovery.

7. It should not surprise us if recovery takes 4,000-plus calories on a daily basis for months. One of the subjects ate 11,000 calories in a day.

8. Dr. Keys and his team found that taking off all restrictions on calories and allowing the subjects to eat as much as they wanted is how they recovered (I found the same thing).

9. We can recover our normal physiology and mental wherewithal, if we eat enough for the body to repair. It will take an amount of time that reflects how much damage has been done by under-eating. Three months did not suffice for men who had been eating 1,560 calories for six months. Patience will be needed.

There are a lot of people referencing the Minnesota Starvation Experiment online, but I think that Doctor Keys would be disappointed if he saw what people are voluntarily doing to themselves that mimics the starvation the young men in his experiment suffered. Dr. Key's wife reported how difficult it was for him to see those formerly healthy young men become weak and sick. He wondered if he should continue with the experiment. As I mentioned, because the restriction the world is engaging in is not a controlled experiment or a real famine, the physical and mental effects that we see now are as highly varied as the individual decisions that people are making about how and how much to restrict. The results are on a spectrum. The ways we are being affected vary and the rate at which we are being killed by our levels of starvation vary too. What should have been known back in 1945 is still being obscured by a complete lack of understanding of the physiology of under-eating and what happens when we start to eat enough again. What healing looks like is misunderstood as a body breaking down, rather than a body building back. It's really too bad, because people are needlessly suffering for too long. We are also inadvertently creating the overgrown fat organs that we are so determined to avoid. We are doing it through under-eating and reactive-eating cycles The Minnesota Starvation Experiment proved that long ago. The reaction our bodies have to starvation is normal. Starvation is not.

Chapter 7

We *Can* Do Too Much

How does exercise fit into the picture of enough calories and good health? As I mentioned earlier, "exercise more" goes hand-in-hand with "eat less", as the most common advice given by those who think they are being moderate. I am making the case that "eat less" is simply bad advice. What about "exercise more"? What about if we eat more and exercise more? Will that be a good strategy for weight loss and make us healthier? It might. It very much depends on what an individual has been doing already.

Exercise does not create energy in our bodies. We may feel more energetic when we begin an exercise regimen, but that is not from the creation of energy. What gives energy to the body is food. Energy has been previously stored in the body from the food we have eaten. If we do not eat food, the body is forced to use its own tissue for energy. If we eat *too little* food, then our body must, also, use our own tissue for energy. A person may feel energetic when the body is using already stored energy from our tissues, but there are limits to how much tissue can be used and allow the organism to remain viable. Eventually, fatigue will set in if food is not brought into the system in enough quantity. The men in the Minnesota Starvation Experiment, spoken of in the last chapter, became emaciated from fat and muscle loss because they were on a strict diet of about 1,570 calories per day. They were walking 22 miles per week and performing some other duties in the laboratory. Their bodies were being forced to operate at a certain metabolic rate, on a certain amount of calories, so that they would lose 25% of their weight in six months. They would have benefited from not walking 22 miles every week on such a restricted caloric intake. They would have lost weight more slowly, but that would not have served the purposes of the experiment.

Moving our bodies is good for us. We are not meant to spend most of the day inactive. The body's immune system is benefited by movement. The lymph fluid, which carries white blood cells throughout the body via the lymph vessels, is moved through the system by our muscular contractions.

Oxygen is delivered to our mitochondria more efficiently when we move our bodies. We maintain muscle mass when we engage in certain kinds of exercise which is a metabolic advantage. If we consistently move our bodies into the full range of motion, squatting, for example, we maintain our body's ability to perform all sorts of tasks as we get older, rather than losing the ability to do these things. But, exercise does not help us to lose fat and keep it off. Why do I say that?

A body will adapt to the exercise and there is nothing anyone can do to prevent that from happening. The body knows how much energy it needs to keep itself in good repair and it will always do the best it can to have that energy available to do the job. In the face of under-availability of energy, it will make all of the adjustments we have already talked about. It will down-regulate the prioritization of certain repairs to certain organs and the production of certain hormones and enzymes and functions of the body in an effort to need fewer calories to keep alive. When an underfed body is being forced to use energy in some way there is less available for optimal function. If the body did not make the adjustments to slow its rate of metabolism, it would have to eat up its own tissue too quickly. This is a life-saving maneuver. What happens if we put physical activity into the equation of too little energy? There is even less energy available to the organism. If someone is under-eating and over-exercising, in the world of eating disorder treatment, this is referred to as Anorexia Athletica. I call it burning the candle at both ends, as the colloquial expression goes. That is how "eat less, exercise more." can get us into dangerous territory. The men who were subjects of the experiment described in the last chapter were eating about 1,570 calories per day and walking about 3 miles per day during the semi-starvation period of the experiment. They were becoming weaker on that regimen. Never can this approach lead to permanent normal weight and good health. We are simply limiting the amount of energy available to the body to perform its basic functions unless we, commensurately, eat more. We will absolutely become more hungry if we institute a new exercise program. If we listen to that hunger and eat more, we will be okay, but too often exercise enthusiasts also institute some kind of eating restriction. They also do intermittent fasting or low-carb eating. They will exercise obsessively, pouring over how many calories they have "burned" during their morning run according to the charts, or consult some kind of activity-tracking device. They will be driven to compensate for that chocolate chip cookie they guiltily devoured, out of pure need for calories, by doing squats until the energy from eating that cookie is used up. What are the results of intense exercise on the organism? Aren't athletes unequivocally healthier than everyone else? Activity is healthful for our bodies, but the answer as to the general health of athletes is not that straightforward. The results of studies talked about below show that athletes are especially vulnerable to certain health issues.

The Canadian Respiratory Journal reports on asthma and asthma medication use among recreational athletes performing in endurance competitions. As the article states, vigorous physical exercise is independently associated with higher rates of asthma, and elite athletes have about three times the incidence of asthma than does the general population[41].

Among American Football players, Alzheimer's Disease and Amyotrophic Lateral Sclerosis (Lou Gehrig's disease) are four times higher

---

[41] Nasman A, Irewall T, Hallmarker U, Lindberg A, Stenfors N: Asthma and Asthma Medication Are Common Among Recreational Athletes Participating in Endurance Sport Competitions: Canadian Respiratory Journal 21 Jun 2018 "we found also cycling and training > 5 h 50 min per week as independent predictors of self-reported asthma. Training > 20 h per week is an independent predictor of asthma among elite athletes, and in a general population sample, training > 2 times and > 7 h per week has been associated with an increased risk of asthma."

than in the general population and neurodegenerative disease, in general, is three times higher[42].

Studies show that Sudden Cardiac Death is the most frequent cause of sudden death in athletes. There is a recent change in how "Athlete's Heart Syndrome" is framed in the literature. In the past it was more often considered pathological. Now, it is considered to be just a group of changes that occur in the heart of athletes as a result of the exercise. It is spoken of as benign or beneficial. As I have already mentioned many times, the body has great powers of adaptation. That does not mean that the adaptations are optimal and will result in the best possible health outcomes. One has to

---

[42] Lehman E, Hein M, Baron S, Gersic C: Neurodegenerative Causes of Death Among Retired National Football League Players: Neurology 2012 Nov 6: "Neurodegenerative mortality was increased using both underlying cause of death rate files and multiple cause of death (MCOD) rate files. Of the neurodegenerative causes, results were elevated (using MCOD rates) for both ALS (SMR 4.31, 95% CI 1.73-8.87) and AD (SMR 3.86, 95% CI 1.55-7.95). In internal analysis (using MCOD rates), higher neurodegenerative mortality was observed among players in speed positions compared with players in nonspeed positions (SRR 3.29, 95% CI 0.92-11.7)....The neurodegenerative mortality of this cohort is 3 times higher than that of the general US population; that for 2 of the major neurodegenerative subcategories, AD and ALS, is 4 times higher. These results are consistent with recent studies that suggest an increased risk of neurodegenerative disease among football players."

wonder if the adaptations, not in the heart structure itself, necessarily, but in the chemical processes in the bodies of those who intensely exercise, result in the higher incidence of Sudden Cardiac Death. Is it just an assumption that the heart of an athlete must be more resilient than the heart of a non-athlete, in spite of the adaptations seen and the fact that athletes are dropping dead on the field? An article in the journal Sports Health published in 2017, reported on studies looking at the incidence of Sudden Cardiac Death in young athletes. According to the article, the studies looking at the autopsies of the athletes who died of Sudden Cardiac Death showed that their hearts were "structurally normal". The journal says that the physical demands of vigorous exercise are what triggered intrinsic cardiac conditions that resulted in the death. I wonder if this is just hypoglycemia. Running out of glucose, which is the body's primary energy source, is deadly. Or is it that the adaptations of "Athlete's Heart Syndrome" are not so benign and scientists are characterizing those adaptations as "structurally normal"[43]?

---

[43] Asif I, Harmon K; Incidence and Etiology of Sudden Cardiac Death: New Updates for Athletic Departments: Sports Health 2017 May-June "Current rates of SCD appear to be at least 4 to 5 times higher than previously estimated, with men, African Americans, and basketball players being at greatest risk. Emerging data suggest that the leading finding associated with SCD in athletes is actually a structurally normal heart (autopsy-negative sudden unexplained death)."

The Female Athlete Triad refers to a high incidence of low energy availability, menstrual dysfunction and low bone-mineral density among female athletes. The incidence of female athletes having no period can be as high as 69%. In the general population incidence is 2-5%. Women with Anorexia Nervosa have an incidence of amenorrhea (lack of a period) at the rate of 66% to 84%. They also have high rates of calcium loss from the bones (osteopenia) just like women with the Female Athlete Triad. What is the message? It does not matter if we simply fail to take in enough energy from food consistently, as with anorexia nervosa, or we fail to allow the body to use the energy, from the food we eat, in the ways it needs to, because we are exercising above what our caloric intake can support. The result is the same in both cases, a lack of energy to support normal body function. The body needs to provide enough hormones for a normal menstrual cycle and it needs to remineralize the bones and not have to chronically draw from them the elements needed to run the body. A body that cannot perform normal functions and stay healthy cannot support another healthy life[44].

---

[44] Nazem TG, Ackerman KE; The Female Athlete Triad; Sports Health 2012 July 4 "Disordered eating---including a range of irregular eating behaviors that do not necessarily meet criteria for severe disorders, such as anorexia nervosa (AN) and bulimia nervosa (BN)---is also fairly common in the athletic community. Up to 70% of elite athletes competing in weight class

There is much resistance to finding anything other than positive results from exercise, so it becomes obvious that researchers are biased when I read the studies. They always begin by saying that exercise is obviously good for us and then go on to report negative findings, while trying to make those seem not so bad. Of course, as I said at the beginning of this chapter, the human body needs to move around regularly.[45] It needs

---

sports (male and female) are dieting and have some type of disordered eating pattern with the goal to reduce weight before competition. The prevalence of clinical eating disorders among female elite athletes ranges from 16% to 47%. The differences in prevalence rates among studies are likely related to variability in the sports studied (eg, weight class or aesthetic sports versus ball games), different screening methods (eg, questionnaires versus interviews), intensity and ages of athletes, and other methodological differences. However, the various prevalence rates of eating disorders in athletes are still in stark contrast to the 0.5% and 10% prevalence among nonathletic men and women in the general population.....Amenorrhea can be caused by......energy deficiency"

[45] Soga M, Gaston Kj, Yamaura Y; Gardening Is Beneficial For Health: A Meta-analysis; Preventive Medicine Reports, Volume 5, March 2017 pages 92-99. "Of the 22 case studies, 7 studies focused on daily gardening and found that those who participated had better health than did non-gardeners, such as reductions in stress and BMI, as well as increases in general health and life satisfaction."

to be engaging in all kinds of activities[46] and be put into all kinds of

postures[47] on a regular basis. Often, the conclusion of a study will say that

engaging in athletics is obviously better than being sedentary. Being

sedentary is not what I am comparing to intense and lengthy exercise. I am

---

[46] Racine E, Laditka S, Dmochowski J, Alamanja M. Lee D, Hoppin J; Farm Activities and Carrying and Lifting: the Agricultural Health Study; J Phys Act Health 2012 Jan 9 "A number of researchers suggest that farmers have a higher rate of physical activity (PA) than those in other professions. Occupational status has often been used in the literature as a proxy for PA, where farm work is categorized as highly physical. All-cause mortality among Agricultural Health Study (AHS) participants, a cohort of farmers and spouses, was significantly lower than the general population; lower rates were also seen for cancer, cardiovascular disease, diabetes, and chronic obstructive pulmonary disease. The researchers suggested that the lower mortality rates may be due, in part ,to the PA associated with farming."

[47] Myer G, Kushner A, Brent J, Schoenfeld B, Hugentobler J, Lloyd R, Vermeil A, Chu D, Harbin J, McGill S; The Back Squat: A Proposed Assessment of Functional Deficits and Technical Factors that Limit Performance; Strength Cond J 2014 December 1 "Fundamental movement competency is essential for participation in physical activity and for mitigating the risk of injury, which are both key elements of health throughout life. The squat movement pattern is arguably one of the most primal and critical fundamental movements necessary to improve upon performance, to reduce injury risk and to support lifelong physical activity.....The squat movement pattern is required for essential activities of daily living such as sitting, lifting and most sporting activities...the back squat can be used to assess an individual for neuromuscular control, strength, stability and mobility within the kinetic chain."

comparing it to living life in a normal way, doing all of the things that people should be able to do. People should be able to walk. People should be able to climb stairs or walk uphill. People should be able to lift moderately heavy objects, like a grocery bag. People should be able to sprint when necessary. People should be able to squat to reach something, lift something from the floor or garden, for example. People should be able to tend to their homes and children and lives without being wiped out or without being on disability at the age of 40. I am not trying to make anyone feel bad if they have been injured, were born with a disability or are quite elderly and cannot do some of these things anymore. I am trying to give a ray of hope, because the things that so many are experiencing in the name of so-called "normal age-related" or occupation-related, or repetitive motion breakdown, are no such thing and it is never too late to repair the problem. We should be moving and we should be able to keep on moving for a very long time. If we cannot, it is due to the body being unable to do repairs through lack of energy in the body that we get from food. If we force the body to do more recreational exercise without compensating with more food intake, it will affect our body's ability to do our normal life activities. We will be too fatigued, for one thing, and too damaged, for another.

We are talking about the ways that intense exercise can impact, in a negative way, the physiology of the human organism, not the least of the ways being, through the draining of energy away from repairs and normal function of organs. If we want to be able to move our bodies in certain ways, we have to feed the body enough to allow all of the usual repairs to take place regularly and all systems to function, as well as enough to compensate for the activity that is requiring calories for its performance. We know that if we drive our car faster, over 60 miles per hour, we consume more fuel and will require more frequent refueling. If we want to run certain functions in the car, like the air-conditioning, we will use more fuel and will have to fuel up more often. We can easily equate the need for more fuel in a vehicle with how we are using the vehicle but, we have an airy-fairy idea of how the human body uses energy. If we want to do more with the body, it requires more fuel[48]. The idea that people have about exercise, though, is

---

[48] Westerterp, Klass R., Physical Activity and Physical Activity Induced Energy Expenditure in Humans: Measurement, Determinants, and Effects; Front. Physiol. 26 April 2013; "Obese women were randomly assigned to diet alone or diet and exercise for 8 weeks. The exercise group participated in aerobic and fitness exercises, in three 90-min sessions per week, supervised by a professional trainer. Daily energy expenditure decreased similarly in the diet group and the diet plus exercise group from 12.3 to 10.8 MJ/d and from 12.1 to 11.0 MJ/d respectively. The PAL was the same for the two groups, before as well as at the end of the intervention. Exercise training did not induce an increase in AEE as observed in subjects with ad libitum food intake. Subjects compensated for the training activity with a decrease in physical activity during the non-training time.....The analysis showed that at the population level, differences in body composition are generally not related to differences in physical activity......at any age, body mass does not systematically differ between a sedentary and a more

that it is how we "burn up" calories so that the calories do not make us fat. We think that we have to do something superfluous to living our life to deliberately use up the calories we consume. We are trying to constantly create an energy deficit. To continue to use our car analogy, what would happen if we created an energy deficit in our car? It would stop functioning, would it not? In this sense the body is not different from a car. Let's consider, though, a way that the body *is* different from an automobile to get some kind of grip on how the body uses calories and how this fits into recreational exercise. This actually illustrates that it is a mistake to view the body in a mechanical, rather than in a physiological way.

I am driving down a country road in my car when, suddenly, the engine throws a rod and I drift to the side of the road with the engine

---

physically active subject......The study included a training program of nearly 1 year in preparation of running a half marathon. Subjects were sedentary men and women who did not participate in any sport like running or jogging and who were not active in any other sport for more than 1h/week... Surprisingly, successful subjects did not lose weight. Apparently, the exercise training-induced increase in energy requirement eventually increased hunger. One has to eat more to maintain the additional training activity, especially in the long term.......Body fat can be reduced by physical activity although women tend to compensate more for the increased energy expenditure with an increased intake, resulting in a smaller effect compared with men. Women tend to preserve their energy balance more closely than men. Women especially do not lose much body fat, even when a high exercise level can be maintained."

banging noisily. What should I do? I have a brilliant idea. I phone a friend to bring a can of gas. I fill it up and leave the car resting on the roadside overnight. I get a ride home with my friend and the next day I come back to find that the gas tank is empty. I fill it up again. The day after that I do the same thing. When I go back again on the fourth day, I top up the tank and put the key in the ignition. The engine starts right up and it sounds fine. I pull out and drive the car without any trouble. The fuel enabled the car to repair itself while it was resting overnight and, therefore, not being required to use the fuel for movement. Where cars are concerned, this is a fantasy, but the body does work that way. I had injured my body by not eating enough to allow it to do small, incremental repairs every night. The quickest route to allowing it to do the bigger repairs that my neglect had made necessary, was to allow it to rest and utilize the more abundant calories I had begun to eat for those repairs. I did not force it to use the energy for extraneous movement, during that crucial time period. I did, however, live my life and do what I needed to do. Now that the major repairs have been made, I can simply eat more when I want to engage in some sporting activity. In the early days, eating more was difficult, for reasons I explained in previous chapters. I mentioned before, but will repeat here, that I built back muscle that I had lost through low calorie and low carbohydrate eating without having to go to the gym. I did not do calisthenics or pilates or anything else. I ate more and especially more carbohydrate to enable my body to stop using my muscle tissue for energy and to build back what my body knew was the optimal amount of muscle for me.

Does the first law of thermodynamics play a role in how a body maintains energy balance? Of course it does. I have heard this natural law used as an argument for the necessity of deliberately choosing a type of movement to utilize calories. The first law of thermodynamics states that energy in a closed system cannot be created or destroyed. The energy can be converted into another form, but the amount of energy in the universe remains constant. In a car engine, the fuel that we put into the fuel tank of the vehicle gets converted into work or heat. If the car cannot be operated, the fuel will stay in the tank and no work or heat will be created from the potential energy contained in the fuel tank. That is why the above analogy cannot happen. In a biological system, however, the energy available to the organism will always be converted to work or heat. We just do not have to deliberately cause it or even be aware that it is happening. A person does not have to say to her body, "I am going to turn you on now, and you are going to work". After an injury, I do not have to say, "I am going to take my body to a mechanic so that he can apply his energy to this damage so that it can work". I might, in severe cases of injury, like a compound fracture, benefit from the work of someone who knows how to set a bone, but let's say that no such injury happens. What will my body do with the energy that comes into the system via the food I eat? It will work on repairing itself. It will use the abundant energy supplied to it from food, during the day, every day, stored in the liver, until necessary repairs are done, often at night. If there is not enough storage fuel, the body will use its own tissues in ways that it must, converting them into the necessary fuel for the mitochondria of every cell. That fuel is glucose. We do not want to stay, for very long, in a state in which the body is forced to get what it needs from its own tissues. That would be like finding that our car had to repair the engine by taking bits from its frame and engine. If that happened to my car healing on the roadside, I would only have to apply extra energy to repairing the frame and engine later, when more energy was available. In the biological organism which is my body, that is what happens when there is not sufficient glucose stored in my liver to do repairs. Now that I have recovered my body's ability to store glucose for the overnight fast, I usually have enough fuel for my body to do what it needs to do. If I do not have enough glycogen (stored glucose), my body wakes me up to eat during the night. This happens less, now, than it did during the first months of re-nourishment.

What we need to recognize is that the body, unlike a car, will always find something to do with the energy we take in, no matter how much it is. If someone has been suppressing their caloric intake for some time, there will be a lot of accumulated damage, so their body will begin using any increased energy availability to do repairs. But, even in the bodily functioning of a person who has never restricted their food intake, their body will keep itself in good repair through the use of the unrestricted energy that is coming in. The person will feel energetic and alert, thanks to this abundant energy. The person will feel emotionally resilient, because there is the energy to keep hormones in production and in proper balance. That person will be able to think clearly, due to abundant glucose reaching the brain cells. Also, the body can waste any extra energy that is not needed, when it is truly experiencing no shortage of energy. A raised temperature is one way that the body will eliminate excess energy. Remember, energy becomes work or heat. Having a normal 98.6 F temperature is a sign of a properly functioning metabolism. Billy Craig, whose year-long 6,000 calorie experiment was mentioned in a previous chapter, gave up the experiment, due in part to being too hot all of the time. Eating 6,000 calories every day for a year did not make him fat, but his body temperature was raised to eliminate the extraneous calories as heat. Eating less allowed his body to stay cooler. He was forcing the 6,000 calorie consumption to prove a point. If he had consulted his natural desire for food, he would not have eaten so much, nor become so hot. His experience illustrates, however, that the first law of thermodynamics is true where biological organisms are concerned. The body will perform work or eliminate the excess energy as heat. It will do those things without our intellectual input. Another way that the body will use excess energy is by making itself fidget. That is why children fidget when made to sit still. We should let them get up and run off their energy. A child who fidgets is a well-fed child. If a child can sit motionless for hours in front of the television, what might that be a sign of? A person may feel like taking on that task that they have been putting off, when their body finally has energy to spare. Their house gets clean and stays clean. Home repairs are made. Maybe their environment is beautified. Maybe they keep their streets clean and plant some flowers, vegetables and shrubs. Maybe they get a promotion for hard work. There is never any need for concern that a consistently well-nourished body will have to store excess energy as fat. The first law of thermodynamics is as true for bodies as for any other system. It is just that we do not have to deliberately apply busywork to "burn off" the energy that we have taken in. Our body will automatically find a way to convert that energy into work or heat. How many of us would like to feel warmer every day? Eating more is the key. Of course, we will also have more fun when we naturally feel like playing a game of tennis. Isn't that better than feeling like we *should* play a game of tennis? A normal, natural and healthy decrease in appetite, without any conscious restriction or suppression will be the result, too, when a healthy metabolism has been restored and the body healed. The formerly much-needed higher caloric intake becomes unnecessary. What Billy Craig's experiment shows is that a person does not become fat and stay fat with a consistently high intake of calories, *because* of the first law of thermodynamics.

What I found out about exercise, in my own case, was that I finally had the energy and desire to move around more when I began eating enough calories. If I wanted to be able to do more, I had to eat more. When I was recovering from under-eating, some rest from the energy expenditure of recreational exercise did me good. For a while, my body discouraged extraneous activity through fatigue. I had to rest more. During that time, however, I was putting on muscle and repairs were being made. If a person is in an eating disorder recovery facility, their exercise will be strictly monitored and curtailed most of the time. That is because it is recognized that the patient needs his calories for weight gain and repair. It is also recognized that exercise is often part of the disorder. Anorexia Athletica is the name given to a pattern of excessive exercise which leads to calorie deprivation. Timing of exercise is also important. Exercising in a fasted state promoted my body's fat storage capacity. For me, that took the form of working for hours before eating breakfast. For others, it is engaging in early morning workouts before they eat.

Sumo wrestlers train to become huge. They are athletes and like to think of themselves as healthy, but the training does take a toll on their health[49]. How do sumo wrestlers eat to accomplish becoming as large as they do? They do "intermittent fasting", otherwise known as skipping breakfast. They train all morning for 5 hours, very intensely, in a fasted state[50]. Doing that will always convince the body that there is not enough food in the environment. When the body has no choice but to use its own tissue for fuel to work out, it will always read that as a signal for fat storage with the next meal. The next opportunity for storing energy comes at lunch, when a sumo wrestler eats a meal of vegetables, meat and eggs made into a soup called Chanko Nabe. They eat this with rice. The amount of calories they eat is usually framed in the media as huge, but it is actually the relatively small number of calories that contributes to their increase in size. They eat, reportedly, only about 4,000 calories in a day, which is not much for those who exercise every day so intensely and whose bodies require high levels of daily repair. It is the injury and repair of muscles during

---

[49] Nishizawa T, Akaoka I, Nishida Y, Kawaguchi Y, Hayashi E; Some Factors Related to Obesity In the Japanese Sumo Wrestler; Am J Clin Nutr 1976 October 29 "Obesity, hyperlipidemia, and hyperuricemia in wrestlers were presumed to be caused chiefly by the high calorie diet and partially by the infrequent meal intake."

[50] Darby, Luke; The Real-Life Diet of a World-Champion Sumo Wrestler; GQ magazine 2015 July 14 "practitioners only eat two meals a day....In traditional sumo training...the rikishi (wrestlers) don't eat breakfast. Mornings begin with a grueling five-hour training session on an empty stomach.....Ulambayar eats somewhere in the range of 4,000 calories a day (not the 10,000 calories as jokingly reported elsewhere)."

exercise that makes them bigger, and sumo wrestlers have big muscles. Extra calories are needed to accomplish that, but they are not getting enough for such a strenuous regimen. The deprivation every morning while they are working so hard makes the body prioritize using some of what they eat later to grow the fat organ. Not eating, while vigorously exercising, is the trigger for the fat storage. Considering that every young man who has never restricted calories needs 3,500 calories to maintain his health and optimal weight, how much would a young man who restricts calories every day need to fuel an intense workout? An extra 500 calories is not going to allow a sumo wrestler's body to repair organs and joints, maintain proper bodily functioning, repair damaged muscle and maintain a fully functioning metabolism and immune system. The sumo wrestler's body is being forced to use energy for the workout on a limited amount of calories, so many things are being down-regulated. Under this circumstance, the sumo wrestler's body is not going to feel it is safe to reduce fat storage. But, getting a big body is the whole point of being a sumo wrestler. This is the recipe for doing that. Keep the body in a state of fat storage by intermittent fasting while also exercising a great deal in the fasted state to force the body to use its own tissue for energy. Then under-eat for the amount of activity being accomplished, so that the body thinks there is a famine. If a person wants a body like a sumo wrestler, this is how to go about it. If a person does not want a body like a sumo wrestler, then they would not do those things.

In the case of the strictly ritual practices of sumo, it is easy to see what is going on. It is easy because it involves a set of established rules. In the case of other athletes, it is harder to completely know what is happening. Linebackers[51], in American football, for example, have practices more difficult to analyze because requirements, of training and body size, vary among the coaches of individual teams. It is true, though, that a young man who dreams of making a professional career as a linebacker for an NFL team is concerned with putting on a lot of weight without exceeding whatever limit a team has set. There is an attempt to put on more muscle

[51] Gonzalez John; It's Totally an Unhealthy Relationship With Food; The Ringer 2020 May 5 "John Greco.....usually played somewhere between 320 and 330, depending on who the coaches were at the time and what scheme they ran. When George Warhop was the Brown's offensive line coach, he favored beefy bodies who could lean on the opposition in the power run game. The year Kyle Shanahan was the offensive coordinator, he wanted his linemen lighter and quicker. He asked Greco to drop about 30 pounds, which he did....there were nights before the weekly weigh-in when he had only a salad for dinner or spent longer in the sauna than usual sweating off water weight.....Greco said. 'I knew a lot of guys that struggled to keep weight on. They'd have to eat ungodly amounts of food. You'd see them the night before the weigh-ins.....some guys would flat out come just to go and they wouldn't eat to avoid a fine. And then there were guys who were eating lasagna, steaks, salads, appetizers, drinks....'"

than fat. Unlike sumo wrestlers, the professional or potential linebacker is encouraged to eat a meal in the morning before the first workout or practice of the day. There is a caloric amount that the player is expected to reach each day. If the player exceeds his top weight allowance, he will be fined. According to the accounts of many players that I have read, they feel uncomfortably full all day, as a result of trying to meet their calorie requirement. In spite of the very high calorie requirement, many linebackers in training are disappointed for some considerable time by not making weight-gain expectations. Some describe, when they are no longer eating this way after retirement, a lack of being able to feel satiated by eating more normal amounts of food. This is how I make sense of how their training affects what happens to their bodies:

1.The player has to be concerned with a weight spectrum of enough but not too much. They eat a certain calorie amount because they think that it will make them gain weight and train so as to create muscle. They may not be allowed to play if they are over a set weight established by their coaches, so they combine eating more than they want with periods of restriction for days or weeks before weigh-ins and games. This is the inconsistent eating scenario that I have described as the real cause of putting on more and more fat over time.

2. However, the difficulty putting on weight, that many potential
line-backers experience, is due to the speeding up of the metabolism that
occurs when anyone begins to eat more. His metabolism will speed up to
match the new level of calories he is eating. The player might lose weight,
unless he keeps increasing the amount he is eating. Of course, if he has
been underweight, his body will use the extra calories, as he keeps
increasing his intake, to increase his weight, by building muscle and
normalizing fat stores. Unless the player begins to convince his body that
the food supply is shaky, by food avoidance, intermittent fasting and so
forth, he will not gain weight. I suspect that the ones who gain, eventually,
are the ones who begin to be erratic about their intake. Perhaps the ones
who find it easy to put on weight from the get-go were suppressing their
food intake before entering the football program. These speculations would
fit with Billy Craig's experience, as well as my own. Any inconsistency in the
intensity or duration of their training, too, can eventually encourage the body
to store some fat. What a linebacker is looking for is a percentage of
muscle mass that is greater than their fat mass. Any person carrying
around a lot of fat also builds a lot of muscle because they are carrying
around an extra load all of the time[52]. The scales begin to tip in favor of fat

---

[52] Cava E, Yeat NC, Mittendorfer B; Preserving Healthy Muscle During
Weight Loss; Advances in Nutrition--An International Review Journal; "The
currently available data in the literature show the following: 1) compared
with persons with normal weight, those with obesity have more muscle

gain and muscle loss when the body becomes convinced that there is not enough fuel for its physical activity. When the body has to dip into its own tissue for energy, it will preserve the fat it has for as long as possible, using muscle tissue for glucose instead. If a player becomes hungry during his workout, it can trigger that effect.

3. A high protein diet is used to try to keep muscle mass high compared with fat gain, but a high protein diet can backfire in this regard when too little carbohydrate is eaten. A high protein diet can have negative metabolic consequences[53]. Excess body fat and diabetes are seen in the same people because they are both symptoms of a body using its own tissue for energy. What prevents that kind of metabolism is eating enough carbohydrates every day. If protein is being emphasized, a player may not be eating the 50% carbohydrate diet that will spare his muscle. Muscle creates a higher metabolic rate than fat does, so the lower rate in a body carrying more fat

---

mass but poor muscle quality.....4) high protein intake helps preserve lean body and muscle mass during weight loss but does not improve muscle strength and could have adverse effects on metabolic function."

[53] Peat, Ray; Glycemia, Starch and Sugar In Context; raypeat.com article "Eating a large amount of protein without carbohydrate can cause a sharp decrease in blood sugar. This leads to the release of adrenalin and cortisol, which raise the blood sugar. Adrenalin causes fatty acids to be drawn into the blood from fat stores, especially if the liver's glycogen stores are depleted and cortisol causes tissue protein to be broken down into amino acids, some of which are used in place of carbohydrate. Unsaturated fatty acids, adrenaline, and cortisol cause insulin resistance."

will favor further fat storage as the body ensures itself against future deprivations of glucose supplying foods.

4. When a retired line-backer no longer has to maintain his enlarged size and cuts back on the amount of calories he is consuming, it is natural that he would feel as if he can never be satiated. His body is bigger than it was and has become accustomed to operating at a certain metabolic rate. Not eating as many calories will cause hunger. The best strategy for taking off the excess fat would be to ease up on forced physical exertion and maintain a relatively high calorie amount on a very consistent basis until the former player's body realizes there is an abundance of calories in the environment for what it needs to do. It is the consistency that is the key to convincing the body that it no longer needs to store excess energy. When the body has adjusted its metabolic rate and repaired itself, the former player will find his appetite becoming more normal. What must always be realized, though, is that these are big men and a 2,000 calorie diet is a starvation diet for anyone, let alone for someone their size. If they are cutting their calories down to these starvation levels, they will feel hungry. Eating until they are satisfied will be the solution. Intellectual judgment about what is a "normal" amount of food will always be wrong.

The strict ritual practices of sumo realize that it takes regular deprivation of calories to create a fattened up body. They consistently create these bodies doing what they do. The exercise training helps contribute to their weight gain by making the body use its own tissue which is the trigger for growing the fat organ in any body. Their excessive workouts mean that energy is being used to fuel the activity instead of being used for many body repairs. Sumo wrestlers suffer some negative health consequences, as a result. Many other kinds of athletes also suffer negative health consequences, as a result of the high energy expenditure which makes it difficult to take in enough energy to compensate for it. In the end, all that I am saying about exercise is what I eventually realized about it in my own recovery from under-eating. What really helped my body heal completely and also grow back muscle that I had lost, was resting and eating enough calories to enable my body to work as it should. When I did normal daily activities or any sporting activities, I had to be prepared to be hungrier and to not ignore the hunger. Hunger is the body's signal that it needs food. That seems so obvious doesn't it? But, if it's so obvious why are we thinking of hunger as a bad thing that needs to be suppressed, either through will power or drugs? Yesterday's energy needs are not today's, especially if I am doing more. To maintain a body with the necessary amount of fat on it and no more, I need to eat what my body is asking for. I never need to deny it anything that it is asking for. As my metabolic rate increased due to the increased caloric intake, my body asked for more food. After my body had addressed the energy deficit and repairs it needed to make, I no longer had to eat as much as I did during recovery. However, each day is different. Moving my body more always requires more calories. Never does anyone have to curtail caloric intake and exercise a great deal to lose weight. Athletes have to be conscious of truly feeding their bodies for their intense level of activity to stay healthy. It is not doing that which causes the health problems they can be prone to accumulate. Very dangerous is burning the candle at both ends and combining intense exercise with under-eating. That takes a serious toll on one's health. Much damage will be accumulated which will be very uncomfortable to repair and take a great deal of time and involve a good deal of pain at times. It is best to adjust our calories upward when we start a new exercise regimen and not say no to our bodies signals for more.

Chapter 8

These Are Not The Enemy

At the age of seventeen, while working at a health food store, I was exposed to the book "Sugar Blues" by William Duffy. From that time on, the complete elimination of sugar from my diet became my goal. It was far from easy to achieve, for reasons I now understand. It took years and years, but I did, eventually, achieve perfection in the avoidance of sugar. During the time of such perfection, I became the most physically debilitated that I have ever been. I had been convinced by "Sugar Blues", that it is the consumption of sugar that leads to health problems. About five years ago, after decades of research, I was convinced that I should add sugar back into my diet. One thing that kept making alarm bells go off in my head about my elimination of sugar was that every advocate of low-carb or no-carb eating that I knew about, developed diabetes while they were eating that way.   Now, I wouldn't dream of eliminating sugar from my diet. Now, I am the most well I have ever been, though I am decades older than seventeen.

There are many foods and nutrients that someone out there thinks should be eliminated from our diets. We have briefly discussed some of these, whether it is meat or carbohydrates or fats, or certain *kinds* of meats, carbohydrates and fats. The most maligned, by the largest number of people, is sugar, by far. It seems that there is a connection between the vilification of sugar and the loss of glucose in the urine when someone has diabetes, in the minds of most people. Apparently, Galen, the ancient Roman doctor, saw two cases of sugar in the urine. Now, there is an epidemic of this condition. What is the reason for this state of affairs? Is eating sugar to blame? Should we avoid sugar so as to avoid diabetes? As a result of reading "Sugar Blues", I thought that sugar avoidance was a good health strategy, for a long time. There are many reasons the body adjusts the blood glucose level higher and a rational explanation for why glucose will end up in the urine, sometimes, when it is. There are processes in the body which are constantly being adjusted by the brain to cope with what is going on. Blood pressure is constantly being adjusted. Blood glucose is constantly being adjusted. Levels of hormones, like insulin, are constantly being adjusted. These adjustments are how our bodies keep themselves in a good state of health or, at least, coping as best they can with what we are doing to them. What is the truth about eliminating sugar from our diets, or any other food, in an attempt to maintain good health? This is a very complicated subject. Many things have been misunderstood and tried. I will explain how I got well. I tried many things over the decades which led to some specific consequences. Many were bad and more recently, they have been good.

There are two stories that started making me think about sugar in a different way than I had for decades. The first is the story of two doctors, from the nineteenth century, who were treating patients who were losing weight and strength fast. They were also losing sugar in their urine. The usual "treatment" for these kinds of patients, at the time, was incarceration in a hospital to ensure absolute sugar deprivation. Those patients quickly died anyway. That is the state that was originally called "diabetes". Dr. William Budd[54] from Bristol, England and Dr. Pierre Adolph Piorry from Paris, France both wrote about their concern that their patients were being tortured by being kept from sugar consumption when they craved it so much. They were dying anyway, so the denial seemed fruitless. To lessen

---

[54] en.wikipedia.org/wiki/William_Budd

their patients' suffering, the doctors prescribed that they be given almost as much sugar as they were losing in their urine every day. A young man, who was Dr. Budd's patient, was given 8 ounces of white sugar and 4 ounces of honey every day. As the amount of sugar he consumed increased, the amount of sugar he was losing in his urine decreased. He gained strength and was able to return to work. The doctor's had other patients they treated in the same way with similar results. The death of one of Dr. Piorry's patients was blamed on this treatment, but it is impossible to say what the truth of it is, from this distance[55]. There was antagonism, at the time, to this treatment, but my own experience of blood glucose rising after I had become perfect at avoiding sugar consumption made me wonder about the experiences of these two doctors.

The other story that got me thinking is the story of hibernating bears. Every year, bears hibernate and while they are hibernating, they become "insulin resistant". Also, while they are hibernating, their blood

[55] en.wikipedia.org/wiki/Pierree_Adolph_Piorry#cite_note-4

glucose rises[56]. When they get up and eat a lot of berries in the spring, their blood glucose levels go back to normal. Every autumn, before hibernation, they have become very, very fat so that they can live off of their fat stores. According to a 2021 article by The Company of Biologists in the Journal of Experimental Biology[57], authored by Kathryn Knight, when grizzly bears hibernate their metabolism drops by 75%. The researchers were wondering about the grizzly which do not hibernate, those who live where salmon are abundant throughout the winter. Could they feed the hibernating grizzly

---

[56] Chazarin, Blanine, et. al.; Metabolic Reprogramming Involving Glycolysis In the Hibernating Brown Bear Skeletal Muscle; Frontiers in Zoology; 6 May 2019 "In mammals, the hibernating state is characterized by biochemical adjustments, which include metabolic rate depression and a shift in the primary fuel oxidized from carbohydrate to lipids....Bears hibernate with only moderate hypothermia but with a drop in metabolic rate down to -25% of basal metabolism.....During hibernation, bears rely solely on body fuel reserves. Fat storage is increased prior to hibernation; e.g. Swedish brown bears (Ursus arctos) achieve this by notably overeating carbohydrate-rich berries....The metabolic rate reprogramming in muscles of hibernating brown bears does involve glycolysis although lipids remain the preferred fuels but with their rate of oxidation being reduced due to metabolic rate depression. Such regulations favor energy savings and the maintenance of muscle proteins..."
[57] Jansen HT, Hutzenbiler BE, Hapner HR, McPhee ML, Carnahan AM, Kelley JL, Saxton MW, Robbins CT; Can Offsetting the Energetic Cost of Hibernation Restore an Active Season Phenotype in Grizzly Bears (Ursus Arctos Horribilis)? J. Exp. Biol. 224, jeb242560. doi:10. 1242/jeb.242560

when they get up every day to fluff up their bedding and cause them to raise their metabolisms and become active? They decided to experiment. The bears at The Washington State University Bear Research, Education and Conservation Center were fed glucose for breakfast over a 10 day period and had their blood analyzed. Their activity levels were monitored for two months thereafter. Quoting researcher Heiko Jansen, the article says that the bears experienced a spike in their blood sugar 2 hours after their glucose meal because bears in hibernation are "essentially diabetic". However, the size of the glucose spike was reducing a little over the course of the 10 day feeding period. This was happening as a result of being fed the glucose. Otherwise, the uninterrupted hibernation of the bears would have resulted in maintaining their normal higher wintertime glucose levels[58]. The fed bears' metabolisms were also increased by 33%. Their activity levels were heightened for almost two months after the 10 day feeding period, as well.

This interested me greatly. In a creature whose normal way of being is to sleep for several months during cold weather, when there are no food supplies, its body makes several adjustments to enable it to keep living.

---

[58] Chazarin, Blanine, et. al.; Metabolic Reprogramming Involving Glycolysis In the Hibernating Brown Bear Skeletal Muscle; Frontiers in Zoology; 6 May 2019 "glycaemia tended to be higher in winter compared to summer...free fatty acid levels were increased during hibernation

First of all, it is absolutely essential that this creature put on a lot of fat to live off of while it is sleeping and not eating. The muscles must be spared, so as not to disable the bear by the time it wakes up in the spring. To accomplish this muscle sparing, two things happen. The bear's metabolism is turned way down to enable it to live off of less energy and the preferred fuel source is switched from glucose to lipids (fats). The bear's cells become insulin resistant to accomplish this switch of fuel source. Glucose is not being utilized as normal. It is being spared for those cells which need it, like brain cells. The animal's muscle cells are using lipids during hibernation. Bears emerge from their dens thinner and ready to gorge voraciously on berries, a source of carbohydrate. As they again eat carbohydrates, their raised blood glucose levels go down, returning to normal. By autumn, they have again become fat, a body mechanism which results from the previous fasting during hibernation. They are now ready for their next hibernation. This happens year after year in bears who hibernate. Their raised glucose levels and insulin resistance are part of the natural process of living off of their fat in hibernation and does them no harm.

Bears spend several months not eating. This is natural for them, when they live in a climate where there is not enough food for months. Hibernation is not natural for humans. If I was going to try to mimic what a bear does when it hibernates, I would spend a lot of time sleeping and not eating. What could I expect from that behavior? When I did start to eat, I would store that fuel as fat because it is the fasting that convinces the body to do that. I will have lowered my metabolic rate, just like what happens with a bear in hibernation. I will have induced the glucose sparing mechanism of insulin resistance, because glucose will have become a precious resource needed for my brain. Glucose levels would be raised, however, as the body ensures that there will be a supply of that energy source for the parts of the body that must have it, deriving it from the tissue in as sparing a manner as possible through the lowered metabolic rate and insulin resistance. However, it must be realized that there will be an elevated blood glucose level because the body will not risk going too dangerously low in this vital fuel for cells, when the environment is lacking food sources of glucose. It will, rather, use hormonal clamps on any excess glucose being as abundantly supplied through body tissue as possible. What would end this situation? Getting up and eating carbohydrate-rich foods like sugar. The Randle Cycle describes the mechanism where one fuel source is used by cells, or another, but not both at the same time. If a cell is utilizing lipids for energy, it will not be using glucose. If the cells of the body are using the fat stores for energy because there is not enough food coming in, especially if there is not enough carbohydrate coming in to supply vital glucose, then many of the body's cells will become insulin resistant to allow the limited glucose to go to the brain and other parts of the body that must have it.

This sparing effect results in the blood levels of glucose being higher, as it bypasses cells on their way to the brain. If I stopped eating every winter, like a bear, and then started eating again every spring, I would be in a cycle of getting fat again. If I was living off of lipids, like a bear in hibernation, I could expect my blood glucose levels to be higher. I will have also instigated a lowering of the metabolic rate.

It seemed to me that what Budd and Piorry stumbled upon was the mechanism for getting out of a situation where the body was eating itself, oxidizing lipids and using muscle tissue to provide necessary glucose and eliminating excess in the urine, because most of the body's cells were insulin resistant. Supply enough carbohydrate in the form of easily utilized sugar, and the body switches from the use of muscle and fat, to the use of the carbohydrate coming into the system. When it no longer needs to use its own tissue, the body calms down and is no longer in an emergency state, trying to keep the brain alive through the catabolism of muscle. I stopped the cycling of not eating followed by reactive eating. I ate considerably more carbohydrates. When I did that, I gained weight for the last time, just like a bear coming out of hibernation and gorging on berries. After eight months of convincing the body that I was not going back into "hibernation", my body started to release stored fat, either detoxifying it and eliminating it in the stool or oxidizing it for energy. It did those things with no instigation from my intellect, completely on its own time table. It did this slowly over the course of years, not months. This seemed to be much safer than the rapid weight-loss diets that I had tried and allowed skin tightening to happen along the way. When I was in a fat-burning period, I could tell from skin issues that would crop up and a feeling of not wanting to eat anything except fruit. I wouldn't feel very hungry, of course, because my body was using stored fat for energy. I wouldn't feel particularly well during that period. Then, my body would end that phase temporarily and I would feel well and ravenous and like eating things that I didn't want before. All of this was resulting in weight loss no matter how much I ate because the body was indicating what and how much it wanted and I was listening. It worked only because I had stopped cycling between eating and not eating. I wasn't hibernating anymore. It is the hibernating in a bear that causes it to become fat during its awake months. That is normal for bears and ensures their survival. For humans, lowering the metabolism to 25% of base is not a normal mechanism. Humans are not happy with the aesthetic results of not eating followed by reactive eating lifestyles. Bears don't mind getting fat and because this kind of life is normal for them, they do not become unwell from long periods of living off of their fat. But, we do.

Reasoning on these accounts helped me to overcome my fear of eating sugar. I thought, "Why would we purposely suppress something that every cell of our bodies needs for an optimal metabolism?" Glucose is the preferred fuel of our cells. If given a choice between oxidizing sugars or lipids, most cells choose glucose. Muscle cells use lipids but existing muscle is preserved through the consumption of carbohydrate, because if carbs are not eaten, the body must convert muscle into glucose for the brain, which is that organ's only fuel. When I had become perfect at avoiding sugar and was severely restricting other carbohydrate sources, I became less well. My blood glucose levels were rising. I was less emotionally resilient. Because I, personally, felt less able to cope with stress, I kept wondering if mental illness was largely due to not eating enough food and especially not enough carbohydrate on a regular basis. Many people are monkeying around with their diet, these days, and many people are suffering mental health issues. The rate at which this has increased in recent years in the United States is alarming. Our brains need fuel and the fuel they must have is glucose. I know, from my own experience, that if I do not eat glucose food sources, namely starches and sugars, I will suffer in many ways. It was adding sugar back into my diet that helped me achieve the complete wellness that I now enjoy. Just like for the patients of doctors Budd and Piorry, my glucose levels became normal again by eating sugar. Any time my body entered a fat-burning phase, of its own volition, for the purpose of eliminating the overgrown fat organ, my blood glucose would be elevated because of the Randle cycle. When that phase ended and my body was not utilizing lipids, I would become hungrier and my blood glucose level would lower again, just like bears experience every year.

All of this is to say that step number one in becoming completely well and losing excess fat stores, for me, was to begin eating sugar. When I began eating sugar again, it enabled my metabolism and digestion to speed up and my intestines to have the mucosal lining they need to be healthy. That enabled me to eat enough calories easily, without having to force it for too long. Step number two was, then, easier, which was eating more. By saying that I eat sugar, I mean that I no longer say no to foods just because they have added sugar. I mean that I started eating anything I wanted, as I have already explained. If I felt like eating milk chocolate, I no longer felt constrained to choose the 90% cocoa varieties. I ate any kind of dessert and have returned to baking, which I have always enjoyed, except during the years when I was telling myself that I couldn't eat sugar. I ate any kind of sweetener except the calorie free ones. I needed my calories to become and stay slim. I ate honey and agave and the less refined cane sugars, but I also ate just plain old white sugar. White sugar and the slightly less refined varieties are 50% glucose and 50% fructose. White sugar is purified using charcoal, to achieve its white color. It is very pure. I let my body decide when and how much sweet stuff I ate. I still do. It has done nothing except return me to the health and slimness that I had before I started trying to eliminate it. When I eliminated it entirely, I became sick and fat. Some low sugar advocates will suggest not eating fruit, as well. I went through that phase, too, in my search for good health. Eliminating fruit from my diet did not give me good health. I think of good, sweet fruit of all kinds as an important element in my return to health and its continuation. Some may feel that if a person allows themselves to eat sugar, they will want nothing but sugar. In my experience, that does not happen. I went through extended periods when I did not want it much. I was following my body's direction, so I went with that. Cookies that I had baked and ice cream that I had bought just sat there uneaten until they had to be discarded. At other times, I really desired a lot of orange juice and other sweet things. I ate cake and cookies and drank smoothies. I drank Coke and Pepsi, too. For sure, because I had so severely restricted sugar sources for a long time, there was a reactive need to eat an abundance of glucose sources at the beginning of my recovery. Sugar is the most easily utilized food that we can eat for energy. It is the most sparing of energy because the body does not have to go through a lot of energy to obtain the energy from it. In a body, like I had, with an energy deficit, it was vital to recovering a positive energy state.

With the mention of Coke and Pepsi, I will address another food category that many feel must be eliminated from the diet in order to achieve good health and a normal weight. My experience of junk food, fast food, processed food, highly processed food, "highly palatable" food, or whatever you want to call it, changed my mind about what kinds of foods can be eaten to recover good health and a slim physique. When my kids were small, they used to embarrass me by repeating to their hosts what they had heard all too often at home. They would call something they had been served as a guest "junk food" and say that they were not allowed to eat it. After one of these episodes, a friend told me something that I thought I would never agree with. He said, "There is no such thing as 'junk food', just 'food'". Of course, I was embarrassed. I told my kids not to turn down what was offered to them as a guest. I did believe that there was such a thing as "junk food", though. Then I experienced my body's cravings during recovery from under-eating. I was learning that it is through cravings that the body tells us what it needs. I became completely well eating what my body asked for, even so-called "junk food", so who is my intellect to argue? My intellect had gotten me into trouble by causing an obsession about the so-called "cleanness" of my food. The expression "junk food" is meant to imply that the substance is devoid of nutrients. I equate that idea now, with how some DNA used to be called "junk". That was a wrong idea. Carbohydrates, fats and proteins are nutrients. They are termed macronutrients. Even a piece of candy is not "devoid" of nutrients, then, if it contains glucose. Are we not aware that when a diabetic's blood glucose level goes too low, a truly dangerous condition, the thing they need most is a piece of hard candy to deliver the necessary glucose quickly and bring them out of that situation that could lead to coma? Under that circumstance, glucose is the nutrient that is needed. If someone has been severely restricting carbohydrate sources, as I had been, that person can expect their body to ask for an increase in food sources of glucose. It is going to ask for them, in fact, from the most easily utilized sources possible, like sweets, a soda or juice, one of those frequently vilified things. As I said before, the reason is so that the body can get the benefit of the glucose without having to expend too much energy deriving it from other things. That brings us to the question, what is "processed" food, anyway?

Humans, unlike any other creature, are optimized for cooked food. The nutrients in many foods become more bioavailable for humans when that food is cooked. Humans have processed food long before the storm of metabolic problems that, as a society, we now experience. We have made beer, wine, mead, whiskey, salami, pepperoni, bratwurst, head cheese, bone broth, jams, jellies, pickles, cheeses, hummus, sauerkraut, bacon, salsa, chutney, soy sauce, tofu, miso, pasta, bread and so many other things. These foods are ages old. These foods are not devoid of nutrients, even though they are processed. Processing is taking a raw, whole ingredient and turning it into something else, like taking a tomato and turning it into a dried tomato preserved in olive oil. Taking a lemon and preserving it in salt and its own juices is processing the lemon. With regard to sugar, it is reported that the juice has been extracted from the cane in India since 4000 BC. For 2,000 years the granules have been crystallized from the juice. Humans derive a great deal of benefit from processing and cooking food, both physical and emotional. It is part of being human. In no way is it the cause of ill health. If we want to think of chemical preservatives and food dyes as a cause of bad health, we could have a case. As an orthorexic, I certainly was concerned about those things before I made my recovery. I won't say that I am unconcerned with unnecessary additives in my food now. The difference is, I experienced my body asking for foods which contained those things, from time to time, and I still became completely well. The body has great powers of detoxification, if it is given enough energy to regularly operate detoxification systems and keep the liver healthy. When I have a choice between food without chemical dyes and preservative and food with those things, I choose the former. I recognize, though, that if a food with chemical dyes and preservatives is all there is, it is better to eat than to be hungry. Not eating was the real problem affecting my health.

The reason for the addition of those things to our foods is for a longer shelf-life and, supposedly, appealing colors. If we would prepare more food at home from the most basic ingredients, we would avoid most of those chemicals. If we would take care to buy foods not sprayed with toxic pesticides, we could avoid those, too. It would certainly benefit our bodies if we could do those things, as much as possible. It is my experience, however, that I still became completely well eating even highly processed food when my body asked for it. When I was recovering from under-eating, what my body needed, more than anything, was calories to address the energy deficit. That was the main element from food that my body needed, at first. It took the introduction of carbohydrates back into my diet to allow my body to begin taking in enough calories, as I mentioned before, however. Remember in the Minnesota Starvation Experiment, the researchers found that supplementing vitamins, minerals and extra protein was of no benefit in helping its subjects recover from starvation (which was eating about 1,560 calories per day) unless they were given abundant food in excess of 4,000 calories per day, ad libitum. At the beginning of recovery, what the body wants more than anything is calories. If those calories come in the form of highly processed food, so much the better, as far as the body is concerned. We can think of a high degree of processing as "pre-digesting" the food. The body has to expend less energy obtaining the energy from that kind of food. That results in net energy gain instead of loss. In the beginning of my recovery, my body surely did want fast food, processed food, and "highly palatable" food. The idea of vilifying food that really, really tastes good is a very strange current trend. Tasting good is what makes food desirable. We need to eat, so food should be desirable.

One of the things that happened to me when I was too picky about every little ingredient in my food was that I limited the accessibility of food to myself. That resulted in an unintentional low-calorie diet. As I said before, I recovered by realizing that it was always preferable to eat something than nothing, as far as my health was concerned.

Does the body become addicted to "junk food"? It is wrong to call anything the body needs in its natural biology, "addictive". There are many substances in so-called "junk food" that the body might need at any given time. It might need calories or glucose or the magnesium in a McDonald's chocolate chip cookie, for example. What happens, in reality, is that at the beginning of re-nourishing the body, it asks for as many easily utilized calories as it can get. Once the energy deficit starts to be addressed, the body begins to ask for other nutrients in less processed foods and eventually, when its powers of digestion are improved, the body begins to ask for more whole foods. It can and will ask for a return to something more highly-processed, from time to time, but those occasions become less. At first, I did not very often want fruit and vegetables in their more whole forms. I had to exercise a great deal of trust, as a former orthorexic, not to second-guess that and force anything. Eventually, my desire for whole foods returned. I started eating apples again, and enjoying them. Apple sauce, apple pie, apple juice, and apple cake with brown sugar icing are still on the table. Everything is. I just eat the form of a food that sounds good to me at the time. I stay completely well and slim doing that.

I used to think that eating a particular food was the difference between being healthy and slim or not. Now I know that the body knows what it needs and it is through cravings that it attempts to get me to eat those things. The more we become capable of denying the body what it is asking for, the more we are engaging in disordered eating. Sometimes the body reacts negatively to a particular food that we want, but that is because our under-eating and especially the suppression of carbohydrate in the diet, has caused us to have some gut issues. If we do not eat enough carbohydrate the mucosal lining in our intestines cannot be maintained. Our guts will become leaky. The result will be endotoxin, autoimmune reactions, gas and bloating. The intestine is trying to heal its damaged cells anytime energy is available to do that work, which is why there is inflammation. The result is an intolerance for a lot of foods. Eliminating these foods will be palliative, but will not cure the problem and the more foods we eliminate, the more difficult it becomes to eat enough calories and get enough nutrients to fix anything. Often we will be unable to comfortably digest grains or milk. The longer the body goes without enough energy to heal the intestines and create the proper mucosal lining, the more prolonged will be the inflammatory problem which makes eating some things difficult. The more my under-eating went on, the more foods I had to eliminate from my diet. There was always something new that I decided I had to eliminate because I couldn't comfortably digest it anymore. At one time, I wasn't eating sugar, fruit, gluten, dairy products, pork, peanuts, potatoes, canned tomatoes, and other things. That was a very dull diet. If I ate too little, I would damage my intestines and enzyme-making ability and would not have an exciting, diverse and delicious diet which would then make it less desirable to eat, which would contribute to the under-eating which started off the whole vicious cycle. Eating more and eating more of the foods that I had eliminated, making myself as comfortable as possible, in the process of slowly reintroducing foods by drinking juices was how I got through the other side. (Some might take digestive enzymes, at this stage.) There is not anything I cannot eat now. I am back to enjoying my meals, especially because they are made up of exactly what I feel like eating at the time.

In my experience, a person will want raw foods sometimes and cooked foods sometimes. They will want more processed foods sometimes and whole foods at others. They will want a hot soup and a cold salad at different times. Sometimes it is the time of year that dictates what the body wants. People have noticed that they want to eat more in the winter than in summer. That is something that should not be surprising or fought against. We do not hibernate during the cold months, as bears do.

We need enough energy to stay warm in the cold. We need optimal hormone production to cope with shorter hours of daylight. If we live in colder climes, we should expect to need heartier foods more than those who live nearer the equator do. One example of how food suited to a climate helps those who live in it is the example of Scottish Highlanders. Bones are sometimes turned up by farmer's plows at the site of the battle of Assaye in India, which was fought in 1803. These bones are bigger and stronger than other bones and are recognized by the farmers as those of one of the men who fought in the 74th regiment of Scottish Highlanders. Those men were renowned for their toughness. Were their bones stronger because they worked harder? Everyone worked harder then. That is not the answer as to why their bone development was unique. They lived in a maritime climate which was very cloudy. It was the same as the climate in Scotland is now. Why were the bones of Scottish highlanders so strong then, but not now? They were not getting more vitamin D from the sun then. Osteoporosis, a condition where the bones become brittle and fragile from loss of tissue, is often attributed to a lack of vitamin D from the sun. What could make up for little sunlight, so that those who grew up in the Scottish Highlands had exceptionally strong bones and not fragile ones? They drank fresh milk and ate processed dairy foods, like cheese and butter[59], and other things that contain natural vitamin D, like fish and offal. (The famous haggis is a Highland dish of offal and oatmeal in a sheep's stomach.) Dairy contains cholecalciferol, vitamin D-3, while butter contains higher amounts of vitamin D-2, ergocalciferol, than other dairy products do. The land in the Highlands is perfect for grazing herds and not so great for growing crops, so the diet naturally developed around available animal products and was what the people needed to eat to cope extraordinarily well with the climate. Are the people who once lived in the Scottish highlands now drinking almond or soy milk and rejecting butter, fish and offal? Perhaps those alternatives are not so suited to the climate of the Scottish Highlands, and do not make a good staple of the diet for those who live in that and similar climates. If so, that might be why bone health is declining. If calcium is not provided from the diet, the body will have to borrow from the bones and teeth when it is needed; like when a baby is being built, for example.

If we reject certain foods on the basis of intellectual considerations, such as the food being too fatty, "fattening", heavy, cooked, processed (like cheese) or because it comes from an animal, we may be rejecting the very

---

[59] Fishman, Stanley A.; The Mighty Highlanders; Wise Traditions in Food, Farming and the Healing Arts 19 July, 2012 "The Highlander's diet was based first on the raw milk of their herds"

things that help us to build a strong body in the climate and other conditions that we must cope with. It requires energy, and exposure to tolerate foods. Lack of energy leads to a damaged digestive tract. Lack of carbohydrate leads to the inability to make the mucous membrane in all of the places in the body it is meant to be, including the digestive tract. Rabbit Starvation is the name of a condition that occurs when we reject fat and carbohydrate in favor of lean protein. It is also called "protein poisoning". When explorers have tried to survive on game meat, like rabbit, the leanness of the meat has caused symptoms of nausea, headache, mood changes, fatigue, low blood pressure, weakness, diarrhea, hunger, food cravings and a slow heart rate. A person could be eating enough calories of lean meat, but be starving. The percentage of protein recommended, generally, in the diet's upper limit is 35%. There is a mechanism in the body for dealing with amino acids that is important to understand. If we eat a meal high in protein without carbohydrate, let's say a burger without the bun or a steak with a salad,[60] insulin will rise to dispose of some of the amino acids. That will

---

[60] Jaminet, Paul; Dangers of Zero-Carb Diets, II: Mucus Deficiency and Gastrointestinal Cancers; perfecthealthdiet.com "I ate a high-vegetable but extremely low-carb diet from December 2005 to January 2008. At the time I thought I was getting about 300 carb calories a day, but I now consider this to have been a zero carb diet, since I don't believe carb calories are available from most vegetables. Vegetable carbs are mostly consumed by gut bacteria, whose assistance we need to break down vegetable matter, or by intestinal cells which consume glucose during digestion."

also clear what glucose there is in the bloodstream. Because there is little to no carbohydrate in the meal, the result will be low blood sugar (hypoglycemia). This state will result in a rise in adrenaline and cortisol and catabolism of the muscle tissue to provide needed glucose. Deciding that it is better to eat just protein without fat and carbohydrate is going to cause problems. The body knows how much protein it needs and will ask for that amount along with appropriate amounts of fat and carbohydrate.

I ate ketogenic diets many times over the years. Ketogenic diets are described by their advocates as high in fat, rather than high in protein. In my experience, however, it is difficult to follow those diets without eating high protein. Fats are not usually consumed on their own. There was only so much bacon I could eat. You have to fill the carbohydrate void with something. Coconut manna is nice, but again, I could only eat so much of that. Four ounces of fatty beef brisket would have 24 grams of fat, but 32 grams of protein. Again, the protein without carbohydrate scenario will put us in a low blood sugar state. Low blood sugar and catabolism is the very essence of stress for the body. When I started to trust my body to tell me what to eat, an interesting thing happened. I wanted a lot of meat sometimes and hardly any at others. Muscle meat, especially, is a more intermittent protein food that I desire. Soups, with their glycine-rich broths, are more often wanted. I definitely do not eat as much protein as I did on any ketogenic diet. I don't necessarily eat muscle meat every day. I do desire more of it, though, than the zero I ate on an ovo/lacto vegetarian diet. I know that many, who are eating a vegetarian diet, dream of steak. I also know that many who follow ketogenic diets, dream of eating cake. The dreams are, literally, the body talking to the adherents of those diets and asking them to address the nutrient deficiencies that they are experiencing. People who have taken up a new extreme diet often feel better for a while. As an example, if someone went from a ketogenic diet to a vegan diet, that person may truly feel better on their new diet. That is because it is addressing nutrient deficiencies that the person had accumulated on the previous regimen. Eventually though, other nutrient deficiencies will crop up on the new diet. The individual will begin to feel less well. If that person then switched back to the original diet, they would, again, begin to feel better as the current deficiencies were addressed. That is because none of those diets are as robust as they should be. Key nutrients are missing because there are foods that are considered taboo in the regimen of each. I discovered that not making any rules about what I ate and listening to my body's desires kept all nutrients consistently available to me.

To illustrate the point I made above, about how the body lets its needs be known, I had a night, recently, when I woke up knowing that I was not going to go back to sleep unless I ate something. I tried to think of what I needed, and decided to eat a poached pear that I had made with some vanilla gelato. I ate that, but it seemed unsatisfying. While sitting in bed, still wide awake, I had a sudden picture of myself guzzling down a glass of milk. What is odd about that is that I never drink milk straight. I combine it with orange juice for an Orange Julius-type drink or make a smoothie or cappuccino or milkshake. Since I was a kid, I have never liked drinking straight milk. However, that is what I seemed to want at that moment, for the first time, ever. So, I got up and poured myself a glass of milk and drank it down. When I went back to bed, I fell right back to sleep. Interestingly, previous to that night, I had been ignoring a symptom that I was having of calcium deficiency. That was neuromuscular excitability. I was having a tingling sensation around my mouth for a couple of days and my tongue was tingling, too. There could be any number of reasons as to why I needed more calcium at the time, and I was desiring more milk products, like cheese sauce and so on, but apparently my body was telling me to up the ante calcium-wise with that glass of milk. I haven't had any tingling since I drank that milk. I have been having more cappuccinos since then, though, with half milk instead of my usual coffee with cream.

This is an example of how the body tells a person that it needs something. With regard to the macronutrients, it works by naturally moving a person, in my experience, to eat a 50%, or more, carbohydrate diet, with protein being right around the 35% recommended. By protein, I mean all of its varied sources, like milk and milk products, bone broth, potatoes, mushrooms, beans, eggs, semolina pasta and smaller amounts of muscle meat than I used to eat. I would be surprised if most people did not fall into something close to those ranges if they were following what their bodies were telling them to eat. As mentioned previously, these percentages may be slightly adjusted, naturally, for climate and other factors. I have never had to purposely manipulate the percentages to achieve a good nutritional status, since I began following my body's indications of what to eat.

Of course, there might be periods when a body asks for more of one thing than it has needed before. A well-fed body will fix long-standing problems when the energy is there and that may require a mineral or vitamin that is in short supply. The result may be a sudden craving for a food that supplies that missing element. Of course, the body can only fix its nutrient deficiencies when the diet is varied and not too rigidly adhered to. What I now realize was so dangerous about intellectualizing food intake, was that I was guessing about and tinkering with my body's needs. I was guessing that a particular symptom meant that I needed to supplement with a particular constituent part of food, but it could have been something else, and it was always a question of how much and for how long, even if I guessed right about what I needed. I guessed and tinkered by adding or subtracting foods and taking supplements in capsule or powder form. I never once felt a sudden craving for iron tablets, even when I was anemic. I might, however, have craved a steak. I never felt a craving for anything in a bottle in the supplement section of any store. Specific food cravings that I have had, however, have been for milk, as I mentioned, cilantro, lemons squeezed in water, a hamburger, cucumbers, mashed potatoes and gravy, apples, orange juice, Coke, cheese like Boursin, black tea, raspberry juice, eggs (soft-boiled, usually), cream soups or cream sauce on pasta, walnuts, peppermint and other things I am sure I have forgotten. There is a lot of variety in the foods for which I have had a craving. The cravings come and go. I am certain that they are telling me what my body needs. I am completely well following the inclinations. Again, never have I craved a vitamin or mineral supplement, only food and drink.

In recovery from the energy deficit caused by under-eating, I experienced the usefulness of all foods. Whether my body was asking for calories or some other element of the food in my environment, it would indicate its need by giving me a thought of food in general and desires for particular kinds of foods. It never led me astray. At no time did any of the cravings I had, for the amount and type of food become out of control. What others judge about the consumption of food by people they know is a real, biological need. Only in the case of someone applying intellectual knowledge about food that has triggered a fear response, do we need to be concerned about someone's food consumption. When anxiety is triggered by eating, or by eating certain things, that is an eating disorder. My cravings were always about the real needs of my body. It took re-nourishment to help me see that I was helped, not hurt, by following the indications that my central nervous system was giving me that I needed something. In learning to trust it, I became completely well in a way that I do not think that I ever experienced before. There is no need to decide ahead of time that I will eat this or that or will not eat this or that. The environment of each person contains foods the body needs. The tragedy is that not everyone has access at all times to enough of what they need to eat.

One of the things that has led to deprivation is the exchange of money for food. When faced with rent and a car payment, the one thing that can be adjusted downward to be able to pay the bills is the grocery bill. If that leads to under-eating, it will have negative health consequences. The temptation is to scrimp on food, even if we have the money to buy enough, so that we can go on vacation or buy an expensive piece of electronics. Most people were better off in the days when they grew and raised a large percentage of their own food. They put up things for the winter and they did not feel as vulnerable as people who have to hand over cash for all of their food. During the recent pandemic, I watched with interest as more people than before, in my lifetime, started vegetable gardens or even started keeping chickens. Why did they do that? Because folks felt that they were in a precarious position. Store shelves and freezer cases were pretty empty for a while. Many started learning to bake. The middle-man supply chain was disrupted and the report was, at one time, that people were not going to be able to get frozen french fries. At the same time, the farmers were dumping their potato crop because their usual frozen foods manufacturing customers were not manufacturing bags of frozen fries because of Covid restrictions. I wondered at the time, why don't people make their own fries? It's easy to do. The fresh produce sections of grocers were not being emptied like the freezer cases were, at the time. Fresh potatoes were there. However, when people have had easy access, for a long time, to foods where the work has been done for them, they do not learn to do the work for themselves. They have been exchanging money for food that has been prepped for them (which is more expensive per pound). They have not developed skills in food preparation which makes a meal's time from kitchen to table faster. One way to lower the cost of food, my favorite way, is to prepare as much as possible from the most basic ingredients. When I walk through a farmer's market or the perimeter of a grocery store, I look at the basic ingredients there, whether it is fruit, vegetables, meats, cheeses and other dairy products and I ask myself what appeals to me right now and what would I like to make from those ingredients. I believe it is necessary for each person in my household to have a voice in what is prepared, since their needs are likely to be different from mine. However, well people are more alike in their needs than the undernourished, and therefore, sick people are. It is sick people who are "all different" primarily, as people like to say. There are a variety of foods in each place on earth that supply the nutrients necessary for health.

That people can be robust and healthy eating a variety of diets was proven by a dentist in the 1930's named Weston A. Price. He traveled the world in search of well-nourished populations eating traditional diets and he found them. He did that because he was worried about the increase in Canada and the United States of dental caries and malformed palates and faces that he was seeing in his practice. What he was looking for, in his travels, were populations of people who were so healthy that they had few or no dental caries and malformations. He wanted to compare them to people, who were related to them, but had moved nearer to shops and stopped eating the traditional diet. He found examples of these groups in the United States among native American peoples, in Alaska among the Inuit, in Switzerland, in the South Pacific islands and among the Aborigines in Australia and the Maori in New Zealand. He also found various tribal groups in Africa who met his criteria, as well as Scottish islanders and people who lived in the Andes mountains. The main thing for each of the groups that he found, who had few to no dental caries and wide palates with room for all of the teeth, which translated to well-formed faces, was that they were isolated from the communities who had access to grocery stores. What Dr. Price found in the relatives of the healthy communities, people who had moved closer to communities where they could be hired to work and where there were grocery stores, was terrible dental problems. Not only did he find too narrow palates with crowded and rotting teeth, but also younger generations of girls whose pelvises were too malformed to give birth normally, mouth-breathing because of under-developed sinuses and a lot of tuberculosis. The data and photos, documenting these findings, are in Dr. Price's book Nutrition and Physical Degeneration. Doctor Price thought that the main problem he was seeing was a lack of nutrients due to displacement of nutrient-dense foods with nutrient-deficient foods. If someone ate something relatively lacking in nutrition, like a product made from refined flour as opposed to freshly ground whole wheat products, the refined flour "displaced" the more nutritious food. I think there is a lot of truth in that, but it is not the whole story.

Here is how I think about what I have read of what Dr. Price witnessed. This is how I think his observations coincide with the story I have told here of my own experience. We are talking about, in this chapter, particular foods and whether we have to exclude some from the diet and include others in order to be healthy, which includes achieving an optimal weight. I agree with Dr. Price that health also includes an absence of dental caries, an ability of teeth to repair themselves when they have been affected by under-nutrition during any period, a proper development of palates and sinus cavities and a proper response to exposure to viruses and bacteria. The variety in the diets he found people living upon in the healthy communities around the world was great. In Switzerland, the people in the isolated Alps ate rye bread and cheese, primarily, with fresh milk and vegetables, in season. When calves were born from their dairy herds there would be veal. Meat was eaten, in general, about once per week. In the Scottish Isles, the healthy populations would eat oatmeal, oatcakes and seafood. In Alaska, those not living on "store grub" ate salmon and each bit of meat would be dipped in seal oil. Because of the extreme climatic conditions in that part of the world, the people had adapted to eat a diet unique from that which the rest of the world ate. For example, they preserved some plant foods by freezing or keeping in seal oil, like sorrel grass, cranberries and other berries, ground nuts (which were actually gathered and stored by mice), and flower blossoms. They dried fish outdoors and the wind would blow bits of sand onto it. This led to an interesting discovery by Dr. Price. The sandy fish would wear down the teeth of the people very quickly. Dr. Price saw that secondary dentin was forming over the pulp chamber in every case where the crown had worn down that much, if the people were well-nourished on the traditional foods. Vitamin C was provided by eating one of the skin layers of a certain species of whale. The diet of the Inuit was a more ketogenic-type diet than any other, because of the amount of fat they ate. North American natives would get vitamin C from the adrenal glands and the wall of the second stomach of moose. The traditional diet was moose, caribou and deer meat, fresh and dried fish, some vegetables and cranberries. Some ate salt-water fish, fish eggs, seaweed and deer. When native peoples in New York kept dairy herds and grew wheat and vegetables, their health was excellent. When the schools their children attended kept dairy herds and grew wheat and vegetables, the children's health was excellent. When Dr. Price visited the South Pacific Islands, he was hopeful of finding people living on a vegetarian diet, but he was disappointed there, as elsewhere. He never found anyone living strictly on plant foods, who was healthy, though he observed groups where a vegetarian diet had been intellectually recommended and was being followed. However, this was not a traditional diet. He reports that he never saw good teeth in those groups. In the islands, he found that seafood was important to the diet, even for the tribes living inland. Wild pigs and coconut crabs were among the important foods. Taro root, vegetables and fruits were also eaten, but not exclusively. In Africa, it was found that among 13 tribes there was not a single person with irregular teeth. The Masai people lived on milk, meat and blood with supplementary fruit and vegetables. Some of the tribes lived on plant foods, mostly, but others also ate fish and had goat's milk. None were vegetarian, because even if they ate primarily plant foods they also ate insects. Dr. Price said that those who ate mostly plant foods ate an enormous amount of plants. Since vegetables and fruits are, generally, low in calories, that makes sense. He also said that while the people in those tribes who lived primarily on meat, milk and blood would be very tall, the people in those tribes who ate both plant and animal foods were stronger and better built. The aborigines in Australia, who lived along the coast, ate seafood, but those from the interior would eat land animals, as well as roots, stems, leaves and berries of vegetation and seeds of grasses. They would also eat beetles and grubs, birds and bird's eggs. Shellfish were important to the Maori of New Zealand who lived along the coast. They also ate kelp and the root of a fern. Where the people continued to put forth the effort to gather those foods, they had very little deformity and tooth decay. In Peru the people developed well on foods including llama, alpaca and guinea pigs, as well as on roasted grains, potatoes, corn, beans and quinoa. In the foothills of the Andes there was fresh fish and tropical fruits and vegetables. The Amazon Forest natives would avail themselves of fish in the streams and animals in the forest. They ate yucca, waterfowl and their eggs and vegetables and fruit.

Since Dr. Price found people so healthy eating all of these various diets that they did not even have many or any tooth cavities, that means the consumption of a wide variety of diets containing different foods, according to one's environment, can contribute to robust good health. Keep in mind that, not only did those populations have few to no tooth cavities, but that state of things was achieved with no tooth brushes, tooth paste, dental floss or dentists. While Dr. Price felt that it was the displacement of less nutritious foods by those that were highly nutritious that was the main factor in the degeneration of one group compared to the other, I think it was more complicated. Those who had come to depend primarily on store-bought foods like canned goods, syrups, refined flours, sugar and jams were certainly displacing more nutritious foods. However, as I said earlier, they were also no longer growing, raising, and gathering their own food. They were exchanging money for food. That always carries the danger of a tendency to under-eat, as money is needed for other things. The diets he describes, of those who were being attacked by dental caries, malformed faces and tuberculosis, were very poor. One boy he describes helping recover health and heal a fracture had been eating white bread and skim milk only. The more we can take our food supplies into our own hands, the more nutrients there will be in our diets. Of course, this also requires tending the soil, by feeding it with organic material and not chemical fertilizers. If we raise our own dairy animals, or buy dairy from local farmers we should be concerned that the pastures are properly managed so that grass is as nutritious as it can be. If we remember, though, the lesson of the Minnesota Starvation Experiment, we will be aware that it was only when the recovering subjects ate enough calories, which was ad libitum in excess of 4,000 calories, that they recovered from the physical and mental ravages of being on a semi-starvation diet (of about 1,560 calories per day for 6 months). The addition of vitamin and mineral supplements and extra protein, according to the researchers, did no good toward recovery until the subjects were given access to unlimited calories. Enough calories, meaning never below 2,500 for anyone and in excess of 3,500 for others, even if they have never restricted calories at all, is of primary importance. Then, the macronutrients and micronutrients can be utilized properly. Certainly, the more one eats, the greater will be the likelihood of obtaining the necessary nutrients. The more variety there is in the diet, the greater the likelihood of obtaining the necessary nutrients. The more ability one has to feed oneself, based on the signals of one's own desire, the more likely the necessary nutrients for good health and a normal weight will be obtained.

Worrying about the micronutrients of food, when I needed to recover from the energy deficit from which I was suffering, was putting the cart before the horse. I was highly concerned about the micronutrient content of my food for many years, all the while getting sicker and more debilitated. In fact, for many years, before I started to understand the importance of calories, I knew about Weston Price's discoveries and had read his book. I followed all of the recommendations of the Weston A. Price foundation, for having a great nutrient status. I did not become well and start to heal, however, until I started paying attention to getting over the 2,500 calories I need every day and stopped restricting carbohydrates. My concern about the kinds of food I was eating was a major contributor to my inability to get enough calories. Preparing all of those foods properly from scratch, the sprouting and fermenting and extra travel for raw milk and so forth, took time. The avoidance of anything like highly processed food meant that I had less access to calories, especially when traveling. Sometimes when traveling I literally starved, out of stubbornness, because I could not find foods that met with my orthorexic approval. When I had access to someone's kitchen, where we were staying, I would bring boxes full of my own food to prepare. All of that intellectual concern did not make me well. As I already mentioned, the first thing my body was concerned with, after I began recovery, was getting all of the easily assimilated calories it could from highly processed food. After some time, I noticed a shift toward more whole and more nutrient-dense foods. Over time, my body addressed any nutrient deficiencies that cropped up because of the repairs that it was making. Today, I have a mostly whole foods diet with forays into highly processed foods. Those foods over time, however, have become less and less appealing. That is because the energy deficit has been completely addressed. Nothing is off of the table, though, and that is the difference from before. If I am hungry, I eat whatever is available and do not prolong the hunger searching for something else. My well-energized body can handle whatever might be in the food by way of preservatives. I always look for food of the highest quality, but I will not go hungry if I cannot get it. This is how I became slim and completely well.

One of the lessons that I take to heart from Weston Price's research is his discovery that the more a group of people relied on vegetable sources of food in their diet, the more of it they ate. He said that the tribes in Africa who ate mostly vegetable foods, plus insects, ate an enormous amount of those foods. As I remarked before, that makes sense when we realize how low in calories most fruits and vegetables are. It would definitely take more effort if I was to decide to eat a vegan diet, just to get enough calories. However, I will not be doing that. In Dr. Price's travels, he continually came across milk consumption in groups of healthy people. In the animal foods is vitamin D. The move to almond milk and such (I used to make my own) was part of the loss of health that I experienced. It was switching to soy milk which initiated my body's intolerance of dairy milk, since it no longer needed to make the enzymes to digest dairy. I eat almonds and almond butter regularly, but displacing highly nutritious cow's milk with almond milk or soy milk was not a healthful move for me. I do not eat a lot of seafood, mostly because I do not live near the sea. I do not care for much offal, either, so I must have dairy products. I eat some of all of those things, but a great deal of dairy. The healthiest of the groups that Dr. Price observed had at least one of those three things as a main part of the diet (seafood, offal and dairy) and often a combination of two or more. As I said before, my body recently upped its milk requirement. The safest way to add nutrients to my diet is to pay attention to what my brain is thinking about. I had been wondering to myself why I had stopped drinking my usual orange juice and milk mixture long before I realized that those conscious thoughts of milk were my body telling me that I needed more milk. I am still learning to pay attention. I have noticed that when I no longer need a particular food I have been eating, I just sort of forget about eating or drinking it. Believe it or not, that can even happen with coffee. When I need it again, I start thinking about it. It is easy in daily life to get so distracted that we do not pay attention to our thoughts, but I have seen how vital it is not to let that happen if I want to keep my body well-nourished. Sometimes the problem that a person has with eating enough is just distractedness and laziness. A regular, iron-clad routine of meals is the antidote to that. It is a beginning, anyway.

The food nature provides is very important. When we have been under-eating for a period, however, we will benefit from "pre-digested" highly processed food to get our energy levels up. That will help us more easily digest other foods that require more energy and enzymes for their digestion down the road. I naturally recovered my desire for micro-nutrient-dense foods as time went on and my digestive tract healed. I did not find it necessary to control sugar intake or any other food in order to become slim and heal from all of my complaints. In fact, restoring sugar to my diet definitely helped my body to heal and eventually eliminate the overgrown fat organ. I ate grains, both soaked and sprouted and otherwise. I ate fatty meat and non-fatty meat, grass-fed and otherwise. I favored non-industrial fats, like butter, over less traditional seed oils. I favored, therefore, saturated above unsaturated fats, and as I did that, age spots on my skin began to fade and are still fading. If unsaturated oil, however, was what there was, I did not reject it and go hungry. I favored whole milk products over low-fat products. I favored wild-caught fish and shellfish over farmed varieties. When I gained strength, I favored homemade over store-bought, but it was the store-bought and fast food that helped me regain that strength. We can definitely be so concerned with quality that it hurts us. I eat the sugar, jam, syrups, white flour, skimmed milk products and canned food that Dr. Price saw the sick populations in his research eating. The difference is that I can, thankfully, obtain the amount and variety of food I need to be healthy. I have, so far, had the resources, so I do not have a limited diet, but rather a highly varied one. I do not exclusively eat less nutritious foods. I eat white bread, yes, but that bread has nut butter or dairy butter and fruit preserves or an egg or sliced meat and cheese on it. There is a lot of nutrition on that bread. And the bread is giving me a great glucose source to energize my body's cells. Of course, the more I eat, the more nutrition I am going to get from my varied diet. I keep, in my environment, as varied a rotating stock of the foods that I feel like eating, as possible. I have learned that it is unnecessary to decide to exclude or include certain foods in my diet, in the hope that those actions will make me slim and well.

I have experimented on two occasions, during the past five years of recovery, with how the Ayurvedic (medical practice of India) food recommendations for the doshas might work with the body's own direction. I have done that because I have noticed that there are some similarities between what my body typically wants and the food recommendations for my "dosha" or physical type, according to Ayurveda. My physical type is Pitta, primarily. That is one of the three main types, the other two being termed Vata and Kapha. The Pitta type tends to get unbalanced, according to the practice, by excess heat, and that is certainly true for me. The general idea is to stay away from foods whose physiological action in the body would increase the character of your own physiology. A Pitta, like me, would stay away, in general, from heating spices, like chiles. Onion and garlic are not used in Ayurvedic cooking, as they are said to contain elements that would increase some aspect of the physiology of each one of the types. They are too "heating" for a Pitta type. I would have to write a great deal about Ayurveda to fully explain it, so I am simply going to explain my experience of following it in an edited version. My Pitta dosha is recommended to avoid coffee and, really, any hot drink. I do not find coffee or hot drinks detrimental to me when I feel like drinking them. When I avoided coffee, simply on the basis of following Ayurvedic Pitta recommendations, I felt less well. I have had periods of feeling really supported by drinking black tea followed by not feeling well drinking it. I do, often, eat my foods at room temperature instead of very hot. This is a natural preference. I think that flavors are better appreciated at a cooler temperature. It is recommended for Pitta dosha to eat foods at a cooler temperature. However, at times I want very warming foods, like hot, hearty soups. If I try to eat something like a salad of grains and raw vegetables at a time like that, I will get very chilled and feel unwell. At another time, the salad will be something I crave and I will feel really supported by it. Dairy products are considered really good for Pitta dosha, and that fits well with my experience of feeling unwell when I ate no dairy products. The recommendation is for raw milk, but then suggests that drinking it boiled is more digestible. The pasteurization process heats the milk, so what is it according to Ayurveda, that would make pasteurized milk undesirable? I explained earlier that I was intolerant of milk after I had eliminated it for a while. I had to gradually reintroduce milk products. I used raw milk, then grass-fed commercial, then any kind, pasteurized or not. I do not, now, notice any difference in digestibility if I drink it cold or hot, like when I make chocolate milk. Tomatoes, and other "sour" foods are not recommended for Pitta dosha. I do find a slight difference in how tomatoes affect me. If I use canned tomatoes, it has to be in something like salsa, which is uncooked. I do perfectly fine eating raw tomatoes and when I make my own sauce for pizza or pasta out of fresh tomatoes, I feel fine after eating them, too. I am not entirely sure what disagrees with me about eating cooked canned tomatoes. Something in the cans lining? Lemons are not recommended for Pittas, but I have felt an absolute craving for them sometimes. In fact, I have read in articles about Ayurveda that the body will "perversely" crave the things that it is not supposed to have. I completely disagree with that idea. I have experienced just the opposite. By eating what my body craves, I make myself well and feel much worse when I deny myself something I want because it is on some "avoid" list. When I have tried to follow the Ayurvedic principles, I feel less well than I do when I follow my body's principles. Even in Ayurvedic texts, it is acknowledged that each dosha will benefit by eating according to the principles of another dosha during a particular season of the year. So, all in all, the best guide seems to be what the body feels like having. That will be most supportive of the physiology of each individual. I believe that is true to recover from an imbalance in the body, as well. We can feel unwell due to exposures to any number of things in our environment. I have experimented a little with using Traditional Chinese Medicine principles about what I choose to eat. The suggestions are meant to balance an individual. As with any other external metric I have tried, I find that I feel less well if I follow it. If it agrees with my body's inclination, it is fine. If it does not agree, I do not feel balanced. Safest for me has been asking myself what I want, at all times.

I used to be a big advocate for the idea that it was mostly a matter of avoiding certain foods that contributed to good health and an optimal weight. I tried various systems over the years. Some ideas were based on erroneous ideas about what guaranteed metabolic health. Some were based on individual differences of physiology like one's blood type. None of these external frames gave me good health and a stable, normal weight. Intellectualizing the intake of ingredients is going to be full of holes. None of us knows enough about all the constituent parts of food and how they interact with each other to start saying something is off limits, or even to say that our diet should consist primarily of one thing or another all of the time. We can deduce much from Dr. Weston Price's observations about the unhealthy and healthy populations in the 1930's. Those populations do not exist anymore because of the incursions, everywhere, of convenience foods and the death of traditional food ways. There are the "blue zones", where a large percentage of the population lives longer than elsewhere, from which we might learn. However, I find that the conclusions reached as to the reasons why people live longer in those places reflect the researcher's bias. They make assumptions about the healthfulness of certain parts of the diet based on current popular belief, ignoring the fact that the same ingredient elsewhere does not seem to lead to longer life. I have given up the idea of making any rules about what I will and will not eat. Even the idea of a "balanced" diet is based on beliefs that may or may not be true, though access to as much variety as possible will ensure the body has everything it needs to choose from. The belief "everything in moderation" can be dangerous because people are guessing about what is too much to be called moderate. Sometimes the body needs an awful lot of something to achieve healing. When that amount is judged as immoderate, it curtails healing. In my life since recovery from under-eating, I feel not only well, but relieved from the burden of having to think so hard about the ingredients in my food every day. Instead, I enjoy thinking about something else, until my body is ready to eat.

Chapter 9

Extreme Distrust and Unnatural Results

In France, geese are force-fed to fatten their livers. This practice is called "gavage" and results in the foie gras that many enjoy eating. In the northwestern African country, Mauritania, girls are "gavaged" for the marriage market. Men in Mauritania find fatter women more attractive. The ages-old practice of "Leblouh" is still done there to fatten a young girl, between the ages of 5 and 19 so that she can make a good marriage. Having a fat wife signals to a man's neighbors that he is prosperous and able to feed his wife plentifully. At some point, the girl's family invests in her future by sending her to a camp where she will be forced to eat between 14,000 and 16,000 calories every day. How is she forced? The camp is isolated and she cannot escape. Women called "fatteners" pinch, hit and squeeze the girl's toes between a contraption to keep them eating. A very young girl will be expected to eat every day over 5 gallons of camel's milk and about 4-1/2 pounds of pounded millet with a pound of melted butter. The girls do eventually gain excess fat, though some are considered more successful than others at becoming sufficiently large.

Is this practice a counterpoint to the experience of Billy Craig, for example, mentioned in chapter 5? Is it a counterpoint to my own experience of eating more and losing weight? No. I don't think so. I will try to come to the balanced nuance toward which all of these disparate facts are leading.

I believe that what finally allowed me to come to my normal weight is trust. I had to start to trust that my body knows what I need to eat, when I need to eat it and how much I need to eat every day. I now trust that only my body can know any of those things at any given moment. I intellectualized the eating process for years under the forces of my upbringing, my culture and my education; that is what got my metabolism into trouble. If I tried to under-eat all of the time, so as to never give my body the calories it needed, I maintained a slim physique, but one that was having its muscle catabolized for its energy needs and whose internal organs and metabolic processes were failing to be maintained. Increasing debility was the result.

The severe restriction of food intake, such as I engaged in, whether officially diagnosed in a person as Anorexia Nervosa or not, has severe health consequences. Some of those health consequences overlap with the health problems that are claimed for girls who have been "gavaged". The list of consequences for those consistently and severely under-eating are: fatigue and fainting, dehydration, kidney failure, loss of menstruation, pregnancy complications, muscle loss and weakness, osteoporosis, slow heart rate, low blood pressure, and heart failure. That is one extreme....consistent under-eating. One does not stay well. If one gives up the under-eating, necessary energy is restored to the body, one again gains weight and health problems can reverse themselves, as I experienced.

The other extreme is represented by "leblouh", practiced, according to tradition, in Mauritania. If someone can somehow be forced to consume more calories than they want to eat, can more fat be stored than is desirable from a metabolic standpoint? Are health problems reported as a result of this practice? Some of the problems reported by girls who have been fed this way are: feeling so heavy that they can hardly walk, high blood pressure, pregnancy difficulties and heart problems. The making of a linebacker also seems to be an example of a kind of force-feeding for weight gain purposes, as mentioned in chapter 7. As reported by former center Matt Birk, he ate 6,500 calories per day while playing American football. Billy Craig, spoken of in chapter 5, ate 6,000 calories per day for one year. Doing that, he became very thin. The unpleasant symptom of doing that, according to Billy, was feeling too hot.

The middle ground is inconsistent eating, where a person starves, then eats in excess of what the suppressed metabolism has been using, that has been caused by the starvation. The starvation, followed by recovery, in the case of the subjects of the Minnesota Starvation Experiment, is an example of this. I lived in this middle ground, for extended periods, when I was not consistently suppressing my diet and my weight. The body grows the fat organ, in response to the previous starvation period, so it was going off and on diets that caused the problem. The fat gain is necessary for recovery from the starvation period. As in my case, stop the starvation long enough and the body eliminates the excess fat in its own way and time. The trust that I developed, by learning about how our bodies really work, was what enabled me to be patient as my body righted itself. Now I know I can eat as much as I want, of whatever I want to eat, any time I want to eat it, and I will not store extra fat. It was to arrive at that freedom and complete physical well-being that I embarked on the journey of feeding myself enough food.. When I was in the cycle of suppression and reactionary eating, however, I suffered many health consequences, as I have already described. The subjects of the Minnesota Starvation Experiment, both during the semi-starvation period of six months eating a daily 1,570 calories and during the recovery period when they gained excess fat and then lost it again, suffered similarly, though in a much more contracted time frame.

These are some possible reasons for me, ever, to eat beyond what I feel like eating: 1.) When my metabolism has been slowed by under-eating. To speed it up again, I need to eat over a certain baseline of calories. For my age, height and gender, this is 2,500 calories or more every day. Eventually, normal hunger signals will be restored and I can trust my body to signal to me when to eat and how much. I will be aware that I will always need to be watchful about my tendency to slip into under-eating, if the reason for it is an eating disorder. 2.) If I am a girl, born in Mauritania, and I am forced by my family to fatten so that I can make a good marriage in my culture. I do not choose to eat that amount of food. That is why I have to be forced. Left to my own body-driven desires, I would never eat that amount of food. My trust in my body's signals to eat certain things, in certain amounts, at certain times is being destroyed by outside control of my food intake. It is my culture that is forcing over-consumption behavior upon me, just as the cultures of others are causing them to adopt under-consumption habits that destroy their trust in their body's signals. My body would maintain energy balance, naturally, without intellectual input, if it was allowed to do so. The first law of thermodynamics would, of course, apply. My body would turn all energy into work or heat and keep only its optimal amount of fat. 3.) I am training to be a linebacker, as spoken of in chapter 7. The desire for work as a professional football player, and the very great monetary and social rewards that come to those who do so, is a powerful driver for me to do what it takes to gain one of those positions where weight counts. Accounts of those who have trained to be linebackers, inform me that eating will become an unpleasant chore when I have to eat more than I want. It destroys the enjoyment of normal eating. The ability to trust my body's signals for what it wants will be destroyed until I recover it by listening to my body's expressed needs. 4.) I am training to be a sumo wrestler, as mentioned in chapter 7. In the beginning, when the new exercise regimen overlaps with eating more than I had been eating before I began training, there may be some difficulty eating the prescribed calories. However, the major reason I will gain so much weight is the consistency of the formula where I will do an extreme amount of training in a fasted state, not that I will be eating too much for my lifestyle. The calories will not be excessive, considering the extreme amount of training I will do. But, perhaps, at first, 4,000 calories will seem like a lot, if I had been eating less than that before training.

Training to be a sumo wrestler will be different from training to be a linebacker. Linebackers often find that they cannot put on weight, when they start forcing themselves to eat more, because increasing the amount they eat simply speeds up their metabolism. It takes a while of forcing food to a certain calorie amount every day to eventually see weight gains, but there are a variety of experiences among individuals who train to become linebackers. Some find it easier to gain weight than others. That is because methods of training for linebackers and the requirements of various coaches are different. It is not the rigid cultural practice that sumo is. Where the individual who hopes to gain that position on a football team has started from, metabolically, varies, as I am sure it must in young sumo trainees. Some were eating exactly what their body wanted every day, before they began their training. Others were suppressing their food intake, for whatever reason. Those who were suppressing their food intake before they began trying to put on weight, are the ones, I believe, who find it easier to put on weight. If they eat erratically, at all, training while fasted, they will put fat on more easily and keep it on. I believe that those who put on weight easily by eating something like 6,500 calories must first have been suppressing their caloric intake somehow because of my experience and the experiences of others, like Billy Craig. If the players simply start eating a lot, with no periods of suppression or fasted exercise, then like Billy, they will simply speed up their metabolism and get very hot, while losing weight.

Billy was experimenting, so he was not trusting his body signals either, forcing himself to eat. I forced more consumption in the beginning to bring my metabolic rate up, but then started to follow my hunger signals, when they finally appeared.

These are practices which, for better or worse, require the forcing of food intake. Only in the case of number one will the outcome be temporary and lead to health restoration and normal weight. It is necessary, for the restoration of trust in the body, because increasing food intake allows for the return of hunger signals. So, what is really happening with the girls being "gavaged" in Mauritania? Of course, it's difficult to say in every case. Some possibilities are that the family is investing in these girls' marriage prospects, beginning at a certain age, so maybe they were not fed so well before they began their leblouh training. Mauritania is not a wealthy country. It could be that some girls' metabolisms are suppressed when they begin leblouh, in which case their bodies will naturally respond with weight gain. However, it seems that many families begin to "gavage" their girls as early as five years of age, though even a five year old can have a suppressed metabolism. At some period in time, the girls may be sent to a fattening camp, where it is the business of someone who is paid, to get the girls entrusted to them to eat. What happened at home, before the girls were sent to the camp? Were attempts made by the parents, and then abandoned, to get their daughters to eat more? Wherever the attempts to fatten them are occurring, the girls are stuffed beyond what they would ever choose themselves, so the parents or fatteners have a fight on their hands and that may lead to sporadic eating at various caloric levels. This overriding of what would be normal calorie consumption of each individual is problematic because of the possible life-long consequences of the destruction of trust in their bodies. Sometimes, according to accounts, a girl's husband complains that she is skinnier than some other woman who was also "gavaged". When a girl is no longer being force-fed, after marriage, is she still eating at the forced level? Not likely. Does she lose weight, hear complaints from her husband, then eat more than she wants, to please him? Does this create an up and down pattern of consumption, like a yoyo dieter's consumption of calories, as they go off and on diets regularly? That is my guess, based on my own experiences with dieting. One thing is clear, at some point the girls are being forced to eat, just like a linebacker in training, more than they want to eat. If they were allowed to trust their own bodies, they would establish a natural energy balance. They would maintain a normal weight throughout their lives and their bodies would have enough energy to maintain their health through time.

There are two extremes of distrust in cultures that lead to an excess fat problem. The Mauritanian culture where force is applied to a girl so that she becomes fatter than she naturally would be, and the American culture and those influenced by its entertainment and media, who obsess over how thin they think a girl should be, disregarding nature. The one makes a girl eat more than she wants and the other encourages her to eat less than she wants. So, where does the common notion that people eat to excess and that is why there is an obesity epidemic come from? It comes from a popular narrative and backwards understanding of metabolism. It comes from a misunderstanding of what is happening when a person diets and loses weight. It comes from a lack of awareness that all of those diets and practices that lead to weight loss, all but one, are degrees of starving. It is caused by not realizing that weight gain is a rebound effect of starvation. When I was consciously (and sometimes subconsciously) limiting my caloric intake, I frequently perceived myself as eating too much. My body was demanding energy and nourishment through cravings and an agitation caused by catabolizing hormones, in response to low blood sugar. In that state, I could polish off a half-dozen donuts in a short space of time. Of course, feeling negative about eating what I perceived as too much, I suppressed my caloric intake again for a few days, until my body again demanded something for my survival. It is the proverbial vicious cycle. If I had kept eating donuts, with no compensatory suppression, I now know I would have addressed my energy deficiency and started to eat more normally, in good time. I suppose someone is thinking, "A healthy craving would have been for a half-dozen carrots. Clearly it is unhealthy to crave a half-dozen donuts." What I also know is that my body demanded something other than donuts, as it, eventually, needed nutrients that donuts do not provide. What a calorie-deprived body is going to ask for, to fix the deprivation, is something like donuts, because they contain a lot of calories. Carrots would not have fixed my energy deficit. Eventually, however, my body asked for something else through cravings, and I ate enough of that thing to address whatever deficiency needed addressing. It took trust to recover a normal body, when I stopped suppressing my food intake either in amount or type of food. I now know that I can trust my body in its desires for any amount and any type of food, because I got well and lost weight trusting it. Before those things happened, I had to trust the research that I had done. I revisited it over and over to reassure myself that it was correct. It paid off because it is correct.

Nevertheless, at the time before I understood these things, I thought I ate too much. After I had been starving, of course, I would eat a great deal to make up for what I had been missing, once I let myself eat. Is that really such a strange concept? If I brought in a homeless and starving person off the street and gave him something to eat at my kitchen table, would I not expect him to wolf down as much food as I would give him? His reaction to having been starved would seem perfectly normal to us. The reaction our bodies have to being under-fed is not a moral failing. We are being directed by the physiology of a starving body to eat to keep us alive, with the hope that we might take in enough energy to allow the body to return to a normal state. The body knows what it needs. It takes trust not to attempt to override this innate, self-protective mechanism, in the diet culture in which we are living. It takes courage to buck the culture's collective fear of excess fat and trust the body we have, though. We have been taught to distrust, if not hate, our bodies. It takes being mentally ill, and in need of help, to be capable of exercising inexorable control over our body's drive to keep us alive and stick to a diet when it is demanding more food and feared kinds of food. We should not congratulate ourselves for our "self-control" in suppressing our diets. The truly rational thing to do is to give up the diet. If we were truly in a deprived environment, with a lot of other people similarly afflicted, it would be a virtue to not be greedy and hoard food just for ourselves. However, when there's no such actual deprivation, except in our own heads, the unnecessary denial of what the body is saying that it needs is not a virtue. When we stringently override our body's signals for what it needs, the end result will not be good. Is it rational to say to the body, you are breathing too much oxygen or that it is not time for a restroom break, when clearly it is? Neither will the result be good when we force it to live on less food than it is indicating it needs. Even if the famine is real and is caused by circumstances beyond our control, the results will not be good, but we cannot do anything about that. Recovery from an energy deficit will be just as necessary when the food shortage is real as when it is chosen by us. That, too, is a lesson from the Minnesota Starvation Experiment. The mock famine in the experiment was every bit as damaging as the real one caused by the war.

Once I addressed the slow metabolism and peristalsis that I had created through low-calorie and low-carbohydrate eating and intermittent fasting, I started to listen to my body. I eventually gained back normal hunger signals. My body could afford to spend energy on hunger signals, once it was convinced there was abundant food in my environment. I had begun to trust that I could eat as much as my body wanted. I had begun to trust that anything my body wanted me to eat, was good for my body. I had begun to trust that I could eat at any time of day, even if it meant getting up in the middle of the night. This enabled me to fix the insomnia problem that had begun during low-carb dieting and intermittent fasting periods. Eight hours is a long time to expect the body to go without food when glucose sources are being eliminated from the diet. The catabolizing hormone, cortisol, rises with a drop in blood glucose and will wake us up to get us to eat and resolve the issue. In recovery, I realized I woke up because I was hungry. My body was repairing things during the night and needed more energy to carry on with the repairs. Once I ate, I would go right back to sleep. No, I did not wake up because I was thirsty. Someone who has recovered her hunger signals knows the difference between those and thirst. They both signal a body need, but a different one. Telling someone that they are really thirsty when they are hungry is another attempt by others, to override trust in our natural ability to perceive what we are feeling and what we need. Many think it is completely abnormal to have to get up during the night to eat. If so, where did the idea of the "midnight snack" come from? I think it came from the historical fact of something called "the two sleeps". It seems, from written history, that people used to sleep in two segments of about the same length every night. The references to this practice span the globe and only disappear during the 1920s and later. A hypothetical scenario, to describe what people might do, is that someone might go to bed at 8 p.m. and then rise at midnight. They would eat something, talk to family members, do some chores, visit the neighbors, read or reflect on their dreams. They would do these things for a couple of hours and then go back to sleep at around 2 a.m. They could sleep another 4 hours before rising at 6 a.m. Of course, the times would have varied from individual to individual. There is current evidence from a study in north-eastern Madagascar, where there is no electricity, that the people living there still practice the "two sleeps". Other studies in other locales in the world did not yield the same evidence, even though those places also had no electricity. Perhaps due to some other factors than electrification, some people have never practiced dividing their sleep. However, there is evidence that people around the world practiced it for millenia. Maybe, when circadian rhythm is consulted, a person would naturally sleep this way. Maybe, if someone was not exposed to a spectrum of light in the evening that mimics daylight, they would naturally fall into this pattern. Some studies have shown that they do. It is clear that people did get up and eat something around midnight or 1 a.m. for a very long time. Perhaps it is asking a lot of the body to go for 8 hours without a meal, especially when the body is required to do a lot of healing. This information squares with my experience of needing nourishment during the night hours. Knowing this historical reality helps me to trust my body and feel perfectly fine about being awake and eating when other people are asleep. It doesn't happen every night, these days, but I'm not surprised when it does. My liver has become healthier and better at storing glycogen for the night hours since my recovery from under-eating, so sometimes a midnight snack is unnecessary, but there is nothing at all wrong with me if I do need to eat then.

Trust that the organism is rational is what is called for, to stop sabotaging our bodies. Some call this kind of eating "intuitive", and it is. However, "Intuitive Eating" has become a method of weight loss, with rules, in some quarters. True intuitive eating has no rules. It is my experience with

truly intuitive eating that has informed me that I cannot overeat. The trust
that I have gained in my body's need for food has made me less judgmental
toward myself and others. "Binging" is a word that gets used to characterize
someone judged as not in control of their eating. Calling *reactionary* eating
"binging" is judgmental. "Reactionary eating" is a biological need following
the previous lack of food. The body is determined not to let us die, so it
demands the food we need to live. It is far from a moral failing. Especially,
when the "binge-eater" is overweight do we judge them. We seem to be
saying to that person, "you should live off of your fat and stop eating so
much". That is cruel, because that is not how the body works. If it is reacting
to previous starvation, and it is, it is asking for what it needs. In following
the body's direction, that person will get well. If they listen to judgmental
advice and diet again, they will not get well. Another judgmental term
applied to eating what might appear to others to be either an
inappropriately excessive amount or particular type of food is "emotional
eating". This is just another negative term applied to what is really just
eating to address an energy deficit or nutrient need. One of the things that
needs to be fixed in an energy deprived body is hormone balance. When
someone doesn't eat enough food, they feel awful. When someone eats
enough they feel better. I started to feel better when I ate more and ate
more carbs. Should I have concluded that eating when I was feeling like I
needed to and feeling better after I did, was "emotional eating" and that it

was a bad thing that I should have stopped doing? What helped me get better was trusting that I needed to eat without any judgment about what my emotional state was at the time. Low blood sugar occurs when someone isn't eating enough. Low blood sugar makes a person feel weak, emotionally shaky and just awful. What I was capable of eating was what I needed to eat to feel well. The body knows what it needs. One of the reasons I object to "Intuitive Eating" as a label is that one of the "principles" or rules that I have seen listed by its proponents is to cope with my feelings by not using food. I consider this nonsense. I spoke earlier in this chapter about the only ways people can be manipulated to eat in excess of what they need. It calls for powerful outside forces of culture or money. In any other circumstance, a person eats what they need to eat. If a person's resilience in life is being challenged, they absolutely need more nourishment to cope.

Since my recovery from under-eating, I frequently have that feeling that "I couldn't eat another bite" when I have had enough. I'm stuffed. I'm full. I'm replete. Whatever you want to call it, it's a good thing. I remember that feeling from childhood, now that it has returned, but those are expressions that I do not hear very often from others anymore. When I was intermittently starving I never felt that way. If anything, I would make an intellectual judgment that I had eaten too much and then feel worried and guilty about how much and what I had eaten. That was not a body feeling, but a mind one. Now that I always eat plenty at every meal and snacks, too, I always feel full in my body when it says I've eaten everything it needed. I can always trust that the feeling will come. When a person is not starving or intermittently starving they will have that feeling. If they have been starving or intermittently starving, it will come, too, but the body will require more food, to make up for its energy deficit. Only by the force of some powerful external pressure will a person go beyond that feeling of being full and that they "couldn't eat another bite". They will force themselves, or be forced, for economic reasons, career goals and culture. If there are no external pressures being applied to a person, like the torture of the Mauritanian girls, then the amount they are eating is the amount they need to eat to get the body on the right track. If they need to do anything "non-intuitively", at all, it will be on the end of making sure they are taking in enough calories when they have been suppressing their intake. That will be a need until hunger signals return. A hunger signal is the thought of food. When I was consistently or intermittently starving I thought of food all of the time. I watched cooking shows and read cookbooks for entertainment, just like the subjects of the Minnesota Starvation Experiment. Now, I do not think about food all of the time; only when I need to eat or prepare for cooking. I just can't eat beyond that feeling of fullness. It makes me feel sick. That sickness is the feeling that linebackers feel when they have to force themselves to eat a certain calorie amount for their job, but they do not want the food. It feels awful and no person with no good reason to continue eating after they get that feeling is going to keep eating. Of course, it must be recognized that when a linebacker finally succeeds in gaining weight, his larger body will require more calories and that amount of calories will then be desirable to his body. So, the amount he can comfortably eat will change. That will also apply to anyone else whose body is larger than it used to be.

Some people with eating disorders try to get rid of the feeling of fullness by vomiting. Bulimia, as it is called, is eating, often to a "binge"-appearing extent, and then ridding themselves of the food by vomiting or by the abuse of laxatives. I have never spoken to a person who engaged in these practices whose reason was not that they feared to gain weight if they allowed the food to go through the digestive tract in the normal manner. That is the powerful cultural motivation that a person needs to do something that is so unpleasant that they feel they must conceal it from others. Another practice that those with eating disorders will engage in is chewing food and then spitting it out. The reason is the same. They really want food, their body is demanding it, but their culturally-driven fear of fat is causing them to avoid the caloric intake of food. In times and places where days-long feasting was the practice, vomiting was how people were able to participate. That is because people really can only eat so much and stay comfortable. The point is, it takes some extreme measures to circumvent the feeling that we try to avoid. The feeling of having truly eaten too much is a feeling managed by our body to tell us to stop eating. We listen to it unless forced not to do so, unless we are removing our food from our bodies in ways never intended for reasons of culture or fear.

Our trust in our body's ability to maintain a proper energy balance has been destroyed by a cultural combination of physiological ignorance, diet culture, the drug industry and judgments about physical variability and what causes people to eat the way they do. I have been called "brave" for going ahead with the plan to re-nourish myself, because I knew ahead of time that it must involve culturally unacceptable weight gain. I had to keep revisiting the science to keep myself encouraged as the compensatory fat storage increased and the companion condition of edema occurred for months. However, the days when the pounds began to come off and the edema went away were great days. I eat as much as I want at all times, and I have only ever, to this day, lost weight. I have my muscles back. I feel completely well. The very last of the extra abdominal fat is almost gone. No pandemic lock-down has caused me to gain weight. (At this writing we are in the spring of 2022. The reason anyone has gained weight during the pandemic is because they were suppressing their intake before the lock-down). I am glad I learned to trust my body. Culture has taught us to distrust the way our bodies work. We have been told, in so many ways, that our bodies are out to get us. The best thing to do is never to act on any of that information and attempt to sabotage our biology. The ways the body will react to the sabotage are perfectly rational but not the ideal. Our bodies' attempts to save us from the decisions we are making may look like just organisms falling apart, but they are not. They are doing the best they can under energy deprivation. They will do much better when we give them the food energy they need. We can trust that. Never go on a first diet. Always eat what the body is indicating it wants in amount, food type and timing. If we have already dieted, we may have made decisions that have hurt us. I am living proof, however, that it is possible to recover from decades of abuse. It can be easier for some to recover than others. My personal story has not involved any medical interventions as my body has remade itself into what was intended from its beginning. Someone else may need medical intervention as systems that were built to cope with suppressed energy intake are rebuilt to an optimal degree. That doesn't mean we shouldn't trust the process. We must cope with the fallout of what we have unwittingly instigated. Energy deprivation has been the enemy and we can do something about that for our future benefit. One big factor to trust is that we will no longer put on excess fat when we are truly eating enough, no matter how much we eat.

Finale

Things I have learned about achieving a normal weight along with good health, in a nutshell:

1. It would have been better for my health and weight if I had never begun my first diet.

2. Because I had suppressed my caloric intake through dieting, I had to allow my body to store excess fat before it would let it go forever.

3. I had to keep my caloric intake well above 2,500 every day, which studies support as the base calorie amount for my height, age and gender.

4. At first, because of a suppressed metabolism, I had to eat even when I did not feel hungry.

5. When my metabolism increased due to eating more, so did my appetite, making eating enough easier.

6. In time, I could trust my body's hunger cues for when, how much and what to eat.

7. I no longer have to worry about the kinds of food I eat, as my body tells me exactly what it needs to achieve good health.

8. My body gained muscle that had been lost without a program of deliberate exercise..

9. When I addressed the energy deficit through eating enough food, I felt like doing more with my body.

10. My body always found something to do with the energy I was taking in, like healing damage, making me completely well.

11. Maintaining a high caloric intake every day is how I stay at a normal weight.

12. Eating richly of carbohydrate sources is how I gained and now maintain metabolic health and a healthy digestive tract, among other things.

13. Eating enough every day helps me to be resilient in the face of daily stresses.

14. Eating an abundance of calories every day is the only way to a consistently normal weight and good health.

Kelly Jones is an independent health and nutrition researcher from western New York.

Printed in Great Britain
by Amazon

35748346R00121